WAKE UP AMERICA!
OUR HEALTHCARE IS BEING USURPED

GINNY BACHE, AKA VK LYNN

authorHOUSE®

AuthorHouse™
1663 Liberty Drive
Bloomington, IN 47403
www.authorhouse.com
Phone: 1 (800) 839-8640

Published by AuthorHouse 08/05/2016

ISBN: 978-1-5246-2230-5 (sc)
ISBN: 978-1-5246-2228-2 (hc)
ISBN: 978-1-5246-2229-9 (e)

Library of Congress Control Number: 2016912640

Print information available on the last page.

Any people depicted in stock imagery provided by Thinkstock are models, and such images are being used for illustrative purposes only. Certain stock imagery © Thinkstock.

This book is printed on acid-free paper.

DEDICATION

I would like to dedicate this book to all of the patients and all of the staff members that I have had the privilege of serving and knowing.

It is because of my interaction with them and concern for all who will be in similar situations that I write this book.

Americans today need to be more cognizant of what is being imposed on them in the name of "improvements in the system". They then must take action to work with their representatives to "make improvements" instead of being led down a blind path into domination.

And I thank Jennifer Nader, LSW for her encouragement, support and advice throughout the process.

FOREWORD

Long-term healthcare is certainly not something most people are interested in talking about. However with the aging of the baby boomers, it is a topic that begs to be discussed at length. The following book provides an excellent perspective on how the system is currently administered by the payer sources, i.e. CMS: Centers for Medicare and Medicaid. More importantly, the author seeks to educate us about what the reality is for being able to obtain quality healthcare.

Ms. Bache, R.N., B.S.N. has many years of experience in the field. She has served as a nursing facility administrator, director of nursing, private duty nurse, home healthcare nurse, and is a registered nurse with special training in infection control, wound care, and possesses an excellent knowledge of pharmaceuticals and their effects. Her background is rich with experience in all phases of nursing. She has weathered the storms of changes with the payer systems in all of the above venues.

As we enter yet another season for what is to become of healthcare with a presidential election looming, it is important to consider what we want. The healthcare workforce in our country will require increased staffing to accommodate the increased "graying of America". What will make nursing and aide work more attractive for the youth of today to pursue?

Jennifer Nader, B.A., M.A., L.S.W.

INTRODUCTION

We have become too wealthy, too comfortable and far too ignorant of what is happening right in front of us that is going to do us all in.

As time marches on, we lie back and expect the government to take care of us; I mean, really take care of us.

Many have become so dependent on the government monies, programs and what they feel is one's individual right to just about anything. So comfortable in "being taken care of" they have not recognized the problem resulting from this. By being "totally taken care of", we are giving away our rights to be participants in what is supposed to be a democracy.

We are literally letting the government take over. "Who'd a thought" as they say?

Well, **Wake up America** the takeover has started.

CONTENTS

Section one (1)
IT'S ALL ABOUT ME.

I grew up in the 1940s and 50s, in a humble, (poor) environment like so many my current age, but we never thought of the concept of being poor.

We had our good clothes, school clothes and play clothes with one, maybe two sets of each. We ate plenty of vegetables canned by the aunts and grandmothers, homemade cookies and bread, butter and cinnamon sugar served as a treat. Having tangerines at Christmas was a huge treat.

My circumstances were a bit different as my mother had died when I was four (4), my younger sister two (2) and my older sister six (6). My father raised us along with the help of aunts, uncles, neighbors and his two good friends Chet Fisher and Red Matthews. By today's standards, I am sure Dad would have been in jail for child neglect, but he really did a fine job under the circumstances.

I only point this out because we all just did what we were told and expected to do. When able, I began working as it was the thing to do in an effort to better myself and work toward a good future.

No one thought of not working or trying to get ahead (of what, I am not sure), but it was a way of life at that time. I was good at just doing what was expected to the best of my ability and cruising through life along with others. I was destined to become a nurse according to my father and anyone able to add his/her two cents worth. My destiny was before me.

I give you this brief introduction because I feel that most people are the same in this regard. We take each day and do what is expected leaving the bigger things to the powers that be to make laws, see they are enforced and do what is necessary to protect and serve us, the citizens.

As previously stated, I was very good at this, just going along, doing my job etc.etc. But then as I matured and went into the military as a nurse, married a military man and traveled to many different areas, I began to look at other areas of responsibility abutting my comfortable life. I had learned more each day from every area of the health care industry and became engrossed in how distorted it has become from the Florence Nightingale feeling I had initially to the business concept it has developed into today.

I am aware that it takes money and a business model to keep the system running, but not until recently had I seriously looked at the system and how it is being run and developed. I reflected on my classes as I finished up my BS degree. I had a three year nursing hospital school of nursing as my introduction into the profession. We spent many hours in clinical practice learning the importance of patient care. I was fortunate to have worked in many areas of nursing and attended four colleges before earning my Bachelor's degree. At times I found myself acting as an instructor in clinical areas rather than a student because my clinical skills were greater than that of some instructors. Other students expressed concern with lack of clinical experience and the overwhelming amount of book education on the importance of management and paperwork. Their Florence Nightingale feelings of nursing were being drowned out and replaced with management process education. I feel that it is critical to retain the caring aspect if we are ever to have responsible nursing care.

My concerns in this area have not gone without comment. I have written many letters to several politicians with descriptions of care causes for concern, but to no avail. I even wrote two small books as a guide for those who may be in need of a nursing home to alert them to the realities. Then like so many, I got busy in my job and with family and I just mulled over the problems at night but kept going on in the status quo.

As with most things, my job came to an end and about the same time I was made aware of an article published in a well know newspaper discussing the race for Medicare Dollars. I was pleased to see that someone had published an article about the current status of nursing home care. It is an area of great concern for many of us in the field of caring for those in need of rehabilitation or long term care.

The push for bigger pools, art galleries, pubs and the like outweighs the insistence on better quality of care in the nursing units. I know that marketing is critical and the shiny penny attracts the most attention;

the penny is quickly tarnished and forgotten. A well cared for patient and the family members will always be grateful and speak of the kind and efficient care that was rendered.

I had one very memorable incident while working as a nursing home administrator that warmed my heart and validated my thoughts: A family member admitted her brother to our facility as a last resort as it was only one of two in the area that accepted residents on a ventilator. The building looked like an old tenement building and had nothing to make it attractive. After several months, I received a letter from the sister in which she expressed her feelings of absolute horror when she approached the facility. She referred to the building as disgusting and could not believe she could leave him there. After he was settled in she began looking for a "more appropriate" facility returning daily and even more often to assure he was being cared for. Several weeks later, she remarked, the care and kindness shown to her brother and other residents was superb. She had only the highest praise for all the staff members and became a voice for the facility.

We would have all liked new fixtures and fancy amenities for the residents, but we preferred the ability to deliver quality care to the residents.

Through the years I would hear remarks over and over again regarding the lack of care and found there was no solution to improving the quality care using the currently accepted models for care. This has become the norm in the nursing home business. I call it bait and switch: Lure them in with a beautiful home and amenities but no money to staff for quality care.

It is a shame that owners cannot interact more with the residents and families to see and feel what is important.

Section two (2)
IT'S ALL ABOUT THE CARE

I am not an accountant, just a nurse who has worked in the field through so many of the changes and applauded the positive interventions by state surveyors and the need for regulations. Like so many things the government gets involved in it quickly became a takeover. The industry is now dependent on the monies from Medicare and Medicaid to keep the facilities running and thus must follow the regulatory guidelines if they are to be paid.

It all sounds so reasonable. It probably could be. However, those writing the regulations and setting the policy for reimbursement for care are the Congressmen and women whom we have elected. I challenge you to ask your representatives how many times they have been to a nursing home or if they have any idea how complicated the process is for a nursing home or a physician to be reimbursed for caring for one patient.

The facilities are paid to care for the residents/patients. The care is delivered by nurses, aides and physicians along with support staff. It should be obvious but the government has made the reimbursement process to pay the staff a game of skills and chance.

The process changes daily. Just as an example, each nursing home must submit a form called the Minimum Data Set or MDS on each resident (patient). This is a form at least thirty-four (34) pages long and must be completed when the resident is admitted, after eight days, after fourteen days, thirty days, sixty days, ninety days then every ninety days after that. The rationale is that it provides the data to establish and work a plan of care for the resident. Truthfully, it is a complicated process. Completion of the form entails the scheduling a time for the therapists, social workers, dietitians, activities person and nursing to compile an accurate assessment of the residents abilities and then to code each problem area. If something "triggers" as a potential problem area, it then must be care planned. All of this under time constraints and must be submitted precisely at the time scheduled. For reimbursement to be forth coming each assessment must be completed on a specified form and in accordance to the formula devised for each designated area. It is so complicated that a special manual name the RAI* manual was created as the bible of instruction on how to accurately complete the MDS. *

Sound silly? Well this multi hundred page *RAI Manual is the Resident Assessment Instrument; in other words, it is the Bible for completing the MDS. It changes almost daily with pages being removed and added and it is up to the registered nurse MDS coordinators to keep up with the changes. Residents on Medicare (those who have their care reimbursed by Medicare) require an even higher frequency of assessments under the prospective payment system.

To add to the confusion, there are different types of assessments with designated forms for each specific scenario; i.e. to start rehab, to end rehab, if they are in a swing bed (in some hospitals, Medicare allows beds to be designated for other than Medicare Skilled beds. Specific regulations are in place for this) etc. MDS nurses are continually under pressure to complete the assessments accurately and on time.

This will be further ramped up when the new Quality Reporting Program is initiated and the facilities are measured based on the quality outcomes. Assessments all hinge on the reliability of the staff performing the care, their documentation and understanding of what is needed and the accurate reporting of such.

CMS and congressional committees are continually updating/ changing the format and criteria for various areas of each category on the MDS. *Why*? I ask myself. It is assumed that quality care and reimbursement are the positive outcomes of the collection and submission of this data. How can continuously changing of the reporting program improve either?

You may not feel this impacts you, but with all of the monies spent on developing new plans, new forms and new committees coming out of your tax dollars, I would think someone would be asking questions.

Having worked as a nurse since 1959 I moved up to administration about twenty (20) years ago. I actually thought that I might have a better chance of affecting the quality of care as a Director. This proved to be only partially true. It quickly became evident that it would be a long and hard fought battle to deliver what I think is good, even adequate care to the residents.

I continue to support the need for improvement in healthcare, but would like to see it directed toward the patients and staff caring for them, not to form more committees that add insult to injury by creating more paperwork instead of time to care for the patients.

Nurses go into school with a Florence Nightingale attitude and find the reality is paperwork and technology. We have only ourselves to blame for the lack of quality care in our facilities.

First, I believe that the healthcare reform is misnamed; it should be referred to as the payment of healthcare reform, not healthcare reform.

Secondly, I feel that we are so shortchanging the patients in nursing homes and hospitals and that by adding the additional burden of more paperwork with less money for additional staff is totally irresponsible.

It is said that Accepting responsibility means recognizing the "what is" of the situation and then identifying our real options, rather than being hypnotized by the "what should be" and being paralyzed by fantasy options. I believe that our Senators and Congressmen are being paralyzed by the fantasies that are being placed before them.

Third, if all the monies spent on committees, redundant new regulations and opulent features were used to insure adequate staffing, a lot of the problems would disappear. I submit the following as one prime example of regulators vs reality in caring for the patients in skilled nursing facilities:

It is the multipage, multi task regulation regarding incontinence in the elderly in facilities. The truth that no one wants to admit is; the majority of the incontinence is caused by a lack of staff assisting those needing to toilet but cannot be attended in a timely fashion.

This is evidenced by the very real description of a nursing unit in a skilled nursing facility that has twenty-five (25) residents: of these residents approximately sixty (60) percent required total assistance to transfer to the toilet = about fifteen (15) residents. Approximately twenty (20) percent or about five (5) of the residents need to be fed or have assistance in eating. Of the remaining residents from those needing assistance to transfer approximately eight (8) will be total care and need checked and changed every two hours or more.

Each unit is staffed with two (2) nursing assistants and one nurse when everyone shows up for work. Each resident takes approximately (and this is low) six medications. To punch out verify and give each medication figuring one minute each you are estimating two and one half (21/2) hours per med pass. Usually med passes are every four to six hours. This is not including the IV's, various patches to be removed and applied, the blood sugar testing and insulin given, and pain meds administered when necessary.

The nurse is also expected to do all paperwork on new admissions, continually assess residents' conditions, notify doctor and family of changes and follow up on new orders. Time to assist nursing assistants in toileting and resident care is non-existent.

The nursing assistants are responsible for the hands on care of turning, changing, bathing or showering residents as well as feeding and toileting. With twenty-five (25) residents to care for is it any wonder that the residents are not toileted in a timely manner and must resort to putting on briefs and becoming incontinent. Healthcare workers are not proud of this fact, but with the increasing load of paperwork piled on by regulations "to improve healthcare and assure reimbursement" the staff members are haunted to have the paperwork in compliance. The patients and residents continue to suffer because we have gone from healthcare to paper care, patting ourselves on the back when all of the boxes are checked and the documentation looks good. Anyone can check boxes and initial paperwork. Good nurses want to minister to those who need care, but time is a commodity in healthcare and the workers are forced to cut corners to meet the deadlines.

Section three (3)
IT'S ALL ABOUT KNOWLEDGE

Another area of great concern is that the education of staff is nonexistent unless staff takes their own time and initiative to learn more. There is no good time to take staff off the units for education unless it is facility wide to meet regulations and leaving areas of care short staffed. With staffing as lean as it is, overtime hours take precedence over education.

Education of hands on staff is seriously lacking but especially critical in the skilled and long term care nursing facilities. In long term care or skilled nursing facilities there are no specialized units for cardiac, orthopedic, surgical or infectious diseases. This puts the burden on nurses and staff as they are expected to care for whatever comes through the door and meet all the needs of each and every resident. Most nurses are LPN's not RN's and frequently nurses new to long term care as they cannot find hospital positions. Many experienced LPN's have excellent skills and can outshine the registered nurses. In LTC and Skilled Nursing Facilities the nurses are usually new to the nursing field and have no one available on each shift to ask questions of and thus get frustrated and leave the field.

Administration rationalizes these turnovers as poor quality of new hires and the nurses and supervisors have accepted it as the way things are. Hence the circle repeats itself again and again leaving the residents with less than quality care.

Surveyors have been brought up in the same environment and thus see only the very obvious deficiencies in care. The training and directions given the surveyors come directly from those writing the regulations and guidelines for the surveys.

I often ask myself if I am expecting too much. I have two answers to this. The first answer is that if I want to keep my job, I go along with the status quo. The second is no, the care can be much better. For this I get my walking papers. A board member at a former facility told me to keep my mouth shut so I can stay around to do more good. I did not make it.

As previously mentioned, education of the front line care givers is a critical area that is very difficult to maintain. It is even more critical in today's climate with research so vast revealing new diseases and treatments daily. What good comes from it if the information is not getting to those caring for the patients? We must find a way to share this information with everyone involved in the care.

A prime example is the wonderful research that has resulted in medications that lessens the symptoms of patients with Parkinson's disease: the medications do wonders, but very few nurses are familiar with the special way in which these meds must be given. When I began my career in nursing and a patient was admitted with Parkinson's disease it had progressed to the point that they were unable to do anything for themselves. No medications could lessen the progression of their symptoms. They were turned, cleaned and fed until bedsores or other infections invaded their bodies and they died. Today, thanks to research there are several medications that allow a person with Parkinson's disease to lead a fairly normal lifestyle.

However, when a patient with Parkinson's disease is admitted to a hospital or nursing facility it is usually a result of something other than the Parkinson's disease. The treatment is then begun for the reason for the admission, but the symptoms of the Parkinson's disease get out of control because of lack of proper medication administration. Few nurses or nursing assistants are knowledgeable about the specific needs of medication administration and care for the patient with Parkinson's disease.

This is just one example of so many patient illnesses in which the care could be better if the information were available to the caregivers.

So much more is needed other than issuing new penal rules and regulations at the top if we are going to achieve quality care in our facilities. If we are to have quality care we must begin with quality care givers. Structures must be in place to ensure the essential education is available to all care givers. There needs to be a sufficient number of staff members to ensure the care can be delivered. To accomplish this, a pay scale reflective of the enormous job they do on a daily basis is available to them.

Long term Care and Skilled nursing facilities are big business. It is growing into a huge business as the elderly population increases. Like most big businesses and those titled non or not for profit they have morphed into "Executive for Profit" businesses with the folks at the top earning way too much money and those actually providing the necessary primary functions that title the business receive none of the increases produced from their labors.

No business can afford huge salaries for everyone, but when the corporation CEO and CFO, etc., are receiving millions each year and the caregivers are receiving around $10.00 and nurses $21.00 per hour one must ask if it is any wonder that there is a shortage of dedicated care givers.

Just a few examples of the Executive pay for CEOs and other "important" executives of healthcare companies in Ohio range from 1.2 million to 5.3 million dollars. How many staff members could be hired with that amount of monies? These figures can be found on the internet by checking for CEO compensation. A quick look on line at the compensation packages is very enlightening, almost sickening.

In looking at the compensation, the securities and exchange has adopted a new rule mandated by the Dodd-Frank Wall Street Reform and Consumer Protection Act of the Securities Exchange Commission. This is supposedly an attempt at pay for performance being available to the public. My feeling is that it is available for the investors, not to advise the general public of how the executive will profit.

Having received my infection prevention certification in the mid-nineties, I am and have been concerned about the lack of support for proper infection prevention programs in LTC. I was very happy to hear of the new regulations to step up the infection prevention programs. My question is: where will they obtain a staff knowledgeable on the subject and the time to educate everyone if they cannot deliver quality care now?

As the structure is today, it is hard to find time to keep accurate records of the numbers of infections in the facilities and it is a continuing struggle to find time to educate the staff on the criteria for infections and then observe and document the appropriate findings. Most facilities keep logs of UTIs, URIs, eye infections and wounds. But it is just a log that they occurred and not the cause or any follow up information. Fortunately enough, most of staff takes to heart the need for good hand hygiene and tries to ask questions on specific cases to keep contamination down. I keep dreaming of the time when everyone is on board with following protocol and are interested enough in reminding others of the importance of it.

To be able to adequately staff and train personnel always comes back to the issue of money. Perhaps in this area of medical care they look for other models to use that would allow them to have consistent staffing. The models are out there are being presented but dismissed by many because "no one would want to work those hours" or some such thing. I disagree; I believe that most good nurses and aides with whom I have worked would be happy for a schedule of dependable staff with training specific to their area of care even if the times are a little different. They look for anything that will make care better and easier for the team.

To provide the funds to make such a change, maybe they could change some of the eight to eighty five percent of Medicare reimbursements available for capital improvements to reimbursement for true quality care.

Section four (4)
IT'S ALL ABOUT CONGRESS

How can we progress to quality care through the regulatory process the way it is structured today? Where do all these regulations come from?

Let's take a quick look at the leadership of our country. It operates similar to many other countries and organizations; a leader, a group of elected representatives that are divided into committees to address the various areas necessary and then sub committees, lobbyists etc., etc.

Have you thought about the fact that each of our states has two (2) senators = one hundred (100) all together and four hundred thirty five (435) representatives to perform the duties for a country of three hundred twenty three million, one hundred seventy thousand and twenty one hundred residents (323,170,021)? Why do I bring this up? I think about my own district and know that the representative has approximately seven hundred ten thousand folks that he/she is responsible to in this small district. The senators have approximately five million eight hundred and six thousand seven hundred and eleven (5,806,711) each to see that their needs are met.

Congress has **five types of committees** -- standing **committees**, subcommittees, special or select **committees**, joint **committees**, and conference **committees**. House and Senate standing **committees** are permanent **committees** that handle most of the legislative business.

The United States House of Representatives currently has 21 congressional committees; 20 standing committees and **one** select committee. All but **three committees**, the Budget Committee, the Ethics Committee, and the House Administration Committee, are subdivided into subcommittees, each with its own leadership.

With this knowledge and knowing that each member of congress is responsible to be assigned and work on specific committees, is it any wonder that it is difficult for them to have a clear understanding of the regulations they are voting on?

Each member is assigned a committee and must learn the facts as much as possible and then is assigned responsibilities in that committee. Whatever the issue, the member then assigns duties for collecting data to his aides/interns to research and find the problems as well as the solutions to whatever the issue is. Simplified, but I am sure you get the idea.

As in most situations, money plays a very big part as to what can and cannot be introduced into legislation. Since quality of care is abstract deciding on a budget for that is difficult, if not impossible. Therefore the budgets for medical care are based on procedural activities and specific diagnoses.

This sounds sensible when presented in this way. Even simple to understand and follow.

Why then have we evolved into the complexity that exists today and what has it to do with the title. "Wake up America! Our Healthcare is Being Usurped"

I feel that one impediment to quality care is the time and money wasted on the over documentation process for reimbursement. In addition, I expressed concern with the coding system for diagnoses which drives the reimbursement for all areas of healthcare in our country.

It began as a simple way of categorizing the diseases and ailments, but once again has evolved into system that enigma would back away from. I know it will probably continue to go forward, but I do find it interesting that one can lose reimbursement if only one area of the HCPCS code might be omitted. There are so many do's and don'ts with this that can jeopardize reimbursement that it is a real wonder that anyone gets paid. It is even more curious to see how many payments are actually correct from the government point of view.

To add insult to injury I began attending seminars on Physician reimbursement changes for 2016. I could not believe what I was hearing. I have placed the outline of one (only one) of the multitude of classes devoted to the subject. We all think the doctors are wealthy and well paid. If anyone is clever enough to work through all of the contingencies placed on Medicare reimbursement for physicians, they deserve any penny they can get.

Many of the areas left a lot to the imagination. Even the moderator hesitated and acknowledged that the format was not complete and he did not know when all of the answers to questions about the ambiguities would have answers.

I will try to give you a look into the latest updates for Physician reimbursement, the Medicare Physician Fee Schedule, as I have interpreted it.

As previously mentioned, the physician must also use a diagnosis code for each condition the patient is being treated for: i.e. diabetes, heart condition, artery or vein disorder, edema, neuropathy, eye disorders, just like in the nursing home and hospital. That's not too bad, you might say. And I can't disagree except that they have now added so many qualifiers and new requirements that physicians must meet the physician may find it necessary to take additional tests and procedures he/she would not have done, just to assure reimbursement.

This completed, there are still more hoops called value modifiers which affect the reimbursement. They have now devised a scale which bases reimbursement on additional criteria such as the PQRS (Physicians Quality Reporting system use) and even the size of the physician's practice. Silly as it sounds, there is much, much more like the non PQRS reporters (those who do not use their system for reporting) and the group risk score however they decide to calculate it.

What ever happened to treating a patient, submitting a bill and getting paid?

I was closing in on this diatribe when I joined a webinar titled "CPC + Model Announcement". The full title is Comprehensive Primary Care Plus.

Pay attention to this! This is the government's way of overtaking all the aspects of your care; learning every detail of your health conditions, deciding what care is getting paid for all under the disguise of "improving primary care". To insure that everyone is on board, CPC (comprehensive primary care group) will bring together CMS, commercial insurance plans and state Medicaid agencies to provide the "financial support" necessary to make this program work. In other words, there will be only one controller of the healthcare in our country.

My son-in law, a true advocate for my position remarked on the CPC stating "it may be good to have more communication easily available to help with treating patients". I agree that would be great except that if you read the goal for strengthening primary care it clearly states that it is to reduce costs. This along with the aligning of all health care reimbursement systems suggest to me that they will collectively decide on what care will be reimbursed. In plain English; One regulatory committee will decide what care can be covered. Not once is it mentioned that the physician will have a say, only a request to provide care.

On another point, if there is to be greater reimbursement for more comprehensive cases, who will be caring for the routine patients?

I know that there are many who might feel that I am ignorant and paranoid. I am neither ignorant nor paranoid but I feel that we are all a part of a giant shell game in which the only way congress can manage the budget for healthcare. It is next to impossible to easily submit a bill and receive fair payment in a reasonable amount of time. If you feel that this is overstated, please look at the pages in appendix #2. I have included the slides for one (1) and just one of the many webinars presented to instruct the physicians on the requirements for submission for Medicare reimbursement as of February 2016. If that is not enough, go to: https://innovation.cms.gov/initiatives/Comprehensive-Primary-Care-Plus to review the presentation on the new program. I have placed the abbreviated version in the appendix.

Should anyone know any of our Congressmen and women, suggest that they too look at this. Everyone can use the internet and go on line to www.CMS.gov type in *Value Based Modifie*r in the search area and review the education films on the subject to learn what Congress has agreed to in regard to the Physician reimbursement.

I feel strongly that our congressmen are not aware of what they are putting into motion. I further believe that some Ed-Psych majors have been contracted to write the programs to meet what they were told was a need to further develop the reimbursement regulation. It begs to ask the scripters, "What is the purpose of this program and have the congressmen really read and reviewed the criteria and the finished product?" We know how busy they are.

To emphasize the enormity of the duties of the members of congress, I suggest you take the time to look at today's (any day) page of the Federal Register. It is online at www.federalregister.gov. To read the Federal Register written data for all to see is a task not easily undertaken. How are the lawmakers able to digest it all and give reasonable responses regarding important issues?

For the information of my readers, the Federal Register is a legal daily newspaper published every business day by the National Archives and Record Administration. The *Federal Register* informs citizens of their rights and obligations and provides access to a wide range of Federal benefits and opportunities for funding.

It is divided into sections that closely resemble the congressional subcommittees. The comprehension should be evident and my concern as previously noted is that they have an enormous job and time can only stretch so far so they cannot possibly know the complete package of every policy when they are voting on it.

Section five (5)
IT'S ALL ABOUT
THE SOLUTION

How can any of the aforementioned information lead to more positive outcomes in the quality of care?

My proposals are simple;

1. Just start with the basics and then look at what is happening to the patients and staff. And I mean, look at them, and not send them a ten page questionnaire. Comfort and satisfaction can be reflected through their demeanor and positive attitude.

2. Cut out the extraordinary coding and daily changes in what needs to be submitted for reimbursement. No matter how you box and wrap it the over documentation of data is not for patient care plans or improving the care, it is for data collection and reimbursement.

3. I am sure that the very intelligent programmers of today are capable of developing a much simpler but effective system of collection that could remain stable for over fifteen minutes at a time. If we have a simple system that can be used for years to come we can save millions on time, training and paper for all areas of healthcare submissions.

Just think what we can save by eliminating the need for RAC*, CERT*, ZPIC* audits to name a few. The *RAC audit is the acronym for Recovery Audit Contractors. This is a specially appointed group of contractors with the task of reviewing records from nursing homes and hospitals to see how many mistakes in recordation have been made that will allow Medicare to recover funds.

*CERT audit is a bit vague, but again a special group of auditors who test the rate of errors in a facility. If the rate is high, reimbursement may be tagged for return.

*ZPIC audits are the mother of all audits. They are the Zone Program Integrity Contractors. They are looking for fraud and it can appear in many ways. It costs a lot of taxpayer dollars to hire the contractors.

If after reading the above material it is decided that we do need this complicated system for detailing the specifics before reimbursing for care, might I suggest that we follow through and have the system globally in the government. This would compel the congressmen and women submit a monthly form itemizing what they have accomplished before paychecks are dispersed.

See appendix number 5 for a suggested form.

Thank you for reading my presentation of some of the atrocious systems our government has imposed on us. Do us all a favor and contact your representatives and be a part of simplifying the process.

Appendices

Appendix # 1

Examples of just a few of the programs developed and need all to be instructed in for compliance.

This information is to assist you in understanding the enormous size of the CMS Healthcare program.

The few pages below do not even cover a smidgen of the vast number of programs written for and to be followed if one is enrolled in or a practicing healthcare worker delivering care.

It concerns me that no one is capable of keeping up with the changes in just a few of the programs let alone those being initiated on a daily basis. This goes back to The Federal Register which does its best to keep everyone informed. TMI: I believe that is the way it is now identified and it speaks the truth, too much information.

If we cannot absorb it, how can we properly use the information?

1

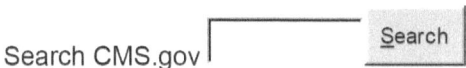

Search CMS.gov

Main Menu

- **Medicare**

- **Medicaid/CHIP**

- **Medicare-Medicaid Coordination selected**

- **Private Insurance**

- **Innovation Center**

- **Regulations & Guidance**

- **Research, Statistics, Data & Systems**

- **Outreach & Education**

Medicare-Medicaid Coordination

Medicare and Medicaid Coordination

- Medicare-Medicaid Coordination Office

Fraud Prevention

- Center for Program Integrity

- How to Report Fraud

- Program Integrity: Medicaid Integrity Education

- Medicaid Integrity Program - General Information

- Provider Audits

- State Program Integrity Support & Assistance

Innovation

- CMS Innovation Center

Provider Type

- All Fee-For-Service Providers

- Ambulatory Surgical Centers (ASC)

- Ambulance Services

- Anesthesiologists

- Clinical Labs

- Critical Access Hospitals

- Durable Medical Equipment (DME)

- Federally Qualified Health Centers (FQHC)

- Home Health Agency (HHA)

- Hospice

- Hospital

- Practice Administration

- Pharmacist

- Physician

- Rural Health Clinics

- Skilled Nursing Facility

Special Topics

- American Indian & Alaska Native

- End Stage Renal Disease (ESRD)

- Medicare Coverage

- Ombudsman

- Open Enrollment

- Partnering with CMS

- People with Medicare & Medicaid

- Privacy

- Program Integrity

- Quality of Care

CMS news

- CMS Blog: CMS Provides Additional Resources to Improve Care and Prepare for the Quality Payment Program for Clinicians

- Fact Sheet: Transforming Clinical Practice Initiative Support and Alignment Networks 2.0

- CMS Blog: Remarks of CMS Acting Administrator Andy Slavitt at the Marketplace Innovation Conference

- Fact Sheet: Pre-Claim Review Demonstration of Home Health Services (CMS-6069-N)

- Fact Sheet: Strengthening the Marketplace – Actions to Improve the Risk Pool

View more news & links

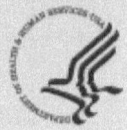

CMS & HHS Websites

- Medicare.gov - Opens in a new window

- MyMedicare.gov - Opens in a new window

- StopMedicareFraud.gov - Opens in a new window

- Medicaid.gov - Opens in a new window

- InsureKidsNow.gov - Opens in a new window

- HealthCare.gov - Opens in a new window

- HHS.gov/Open - Opens in a new window

Tools

- Acronyms - Opens in a new window

- Contacts - Opens in a new window

- FAQs - Opens in a new window

- Glossary - Opens in a new window

- Archive - Opens in a new window

Helpful Links

- Web Policies & Important Links

- Privacy Policy

- Plain Language

- Freedom of Information Act

- No Fear Act

- Nondiscrimination/Accessibility

- HHS.gov - Opens in a new window

- Inspector General - Opens in a new window

- USA.gov - Opens in a new window

2

- **Return to List**

Details for title: 100-08

Publication #

100-08

Title

Medicare Program Integrity Manual

Downloads

- Chapter 1 - Overview of Medical Review (MR) and Benefit Integrity (BI) Programs [PDF, 113KB]

- Chapter 2 - Data Analysis [PDF, 80KB]

- Chapter 3 - Verifying Potential Errors and Taking Corrective Actions [PDF, 606KB]

- Chapter 4 - Benefit Integrity [PDF, 653KB]

- Chapter 5 - Items and Services Having Special DME Review Considerations [PDF, 183KB]

- Chapter 6 - Medicare Contractor Medical Review Guidelines for Specific Services [PDF, 257KB]

- Chapter 7 - MR Reports [PDF, 246KB]

- Chapter 8 - Administrative Actions and Statistical Sampling for Overpayment Estimates [PDF, 214KB]

- Chapter 9 - Reserved for Future Use [PDF, 30KB]

- Chapter 10 - Reserved for Future Use [PDF, 113KB]

- Chapter 11 - Fiscal Administration [PDF, 97KB]

- Chapter 12 - The Comprehensive Error Rate Testing Program [PDF, 109KB]

- Chapter 13 - Local Coverage Determinations [PDF, 219KB]

- Chapter 14 - Reserved for Future Use [PDF, 26KB]

- Chapter 15 - Medicare Enrollment [PDF, 1MB]

- Exhibits [PDF, 1MB]

- Help with File Formats and Plug-Ins

APPENDIX # 2
Physician Reimbursement

A brief look at the program for physician reimbursement.

This is the first seventeen (17) pages of the first module of instructions for the Physician and professionals' reimbursement.

I include this to make you aware of the complexity of the program.

Page two (2) indexes the six modules that need to be completed. It can be seen in its entirety by logging on to www.CMS.gov and going to the Medicare Quality Reporting Programs. They are in the MLN, (Medicare Learning Network).

Each module contains approximately seventy-five (75) pages.

Imagine going through this process just to be reimbursed for doing your job.

That would probably not be to staggering if it were to be the final chapter, but if history will repeat itself; they will make changes in the process on a regular basis requiring continuous reeducation of the updates.

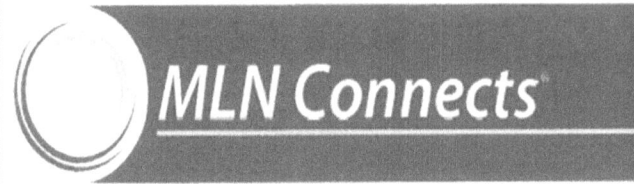

The Medicare Quality Reporting Programs:

What Eligible Professionals Need to Know in 2016

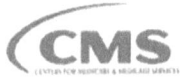

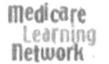

medicare
Learning
network

Official Information Health Care
Professionals Can Trust

Modules

- Module 1: Medicare Access and CHIP Reauthorization Act (MACRA) Preview
- Module 2: 2016 Incentive Payments and 2018 Payment Adjustments
- Module 3: 2016 PQRS Updates
- Module 4: 2018 Value-based Payment Modifier (VM) Policies
- Module 5: Physician Compare Updates for 2016
- Module 6: Meaningful Use of CEHRT in 2016

Module 1: Medicare Access and CHIP Reauthorization Act (MACRA) Preview

Medicare Access and CHIP Reauthorization Act (MACRA) Preview

- Separate application of payment adjustments under PQRS, VM, and EHR-MU will sunset Dec. 31, 2018
- January 1, 2019 – Merit-Based Incentive Payment System (MIPS) and Alternative Payment Model (APM) incentive payments begin
- EPs can participate in MIPS or meet requirements to be qualifying APM participant
- MIPS – Can receive positive, negative or zero payment adjustment
- APM Participant – If criteria are met, can receive 5 percent incentive payment for 6 years

Medicare Access and CHIP Reauthorization Act (MACRA) Preview: MIPS

- Applies to individual EPs, groups of EPs or virtual groups
- 2019 & 2020 (First two years)
  - Physicians, PAs
  - Certified Registered Nurse Anesthetists
  - NPs, Clinical Nurse Specialists
  - Groups that include such professionals
- 2021 onward
  - Secretary can add EPs (described in 1848(k)(3)(B)) to MIPS
- Excluded EPs
  - Qualifying APM participants (QP)
  - Partial Qualifying APM Participants
  - Low volume threshold exclusions

Medicare Access and CHIP Reauthorization Act (MACRA) Preview: MIPS

Year	Performance Categories				MIPS Adjustment Factor (+/-)
	Quality Measures	Resource Use	Clinical Improvement Activities	Meaningful Use of Certified EHR Technology	
2019	50%	10%	15%	25%	+/- 4%
2020	45%	15%	15%	25%	+/- 5%
2021	30%	30%	15%	25%	+/- 7%
2022 and beyond	30%	30%	15%	25%	+/- 9%

- The composite performance score will range from 0 – 100

- Statute establishes formula for calculating payment adjustment factors relative to performance threshold and established "applicable percent" amounts.

- EPs receive a positive adjustment factor if score is above the performance threshold and a negative adjustment factor if score is below threshold.

Module 2: 2016 Incentive Payments and 2018 Payment Adjustments

Medicare Access and CHIP Reauthorization Act (MACRA) Preview: APMs

- Beginning in 2019 and for 6 years 5% incentive payment for:
  - EPs or groups of EPs who participate in certain types of APMs and who meet specified payment amount or patient count thresholds.
  - Payment is made in a lump sum on an annual basis.
  - EPs or groups of EPs meeting criteria to receive APM incentive payment are excluded from the requirements of MIPS.

- To earn the incentive payment, an EP must participate in an APM that meets the following criteria :
  - Requires participants to use certified EHR technology
  - Provides payment for covered professional services based on quality measures "comparable to" MIPS quality measures; AND
  - Either:

    (a) Entities participating in the APM bear financial risk for monetary losses that are in excess of a nominal amount; OR

    (b) APM is a medical home model expanded under section 1115A(c) of the SSA.

Module 2: 2016 Incentive Payments and 2018 Payment Adjustments

2016 Incentive Payments and 2018 Payment Adjustments

	PQRS	Value Modifier						EHR Incentive Program			
		Groups with 2-9 EPs & Solo Practitioners			Groups with 10+ EPs						
	Pay Adj (2018)	PQRS-Reporting (Up or Neutral Adj) (2018)	PQRS-Reporting (Down Adj) (2018)	Non PQRS Reporting (2018)	PQRS-Reporting (Up or Neutral Adj) (2018)	PQRS-Reporting (Down Adj) (2018)	Non PQRS Reporting (2018)	Medicare Inc. (2016)	Medicaid Inc. (2016)	Medicare Pay Adj (2018)	Total Medicare Payment Adjustments or Risk for Non Participation FOR EHR Meaningful Use 2018
Physicians											
MD & DO	-2.0% of MPFS	+2.0 (x), +1.0(x), or neutral	-1.0% or 2.0% of MPFS	-2.0% of MPFS	+4.0 (x), +2.0(x), or neutral	2.0% or -4.0% of MPFS	-4.0% of MPFS	$2,000-$4,000 (based on when EP 1st demo MU)	$8,500 or $21,250 (based on when EP did A/I/U)	-3.0% of MPFS	Physicians in groups of 2-9 EPs & Solo physicians -2.0%
DDM											
Oral Sur									N/A		Physicians in groups of 10+ EPs -3.0%
Pod.											
Opt.											
Chiro.											

9

	PQRS	Value Modifier									EHR			Total Medicare Payment Adjustments which for Non-Physicians in PQRS and Meaningful Use in 2018
			Groups with Non-Physician EPs only and Solo Practitioners	Groups with Physicians + PAs, NPs, CNSs, & CRNAs								Medicare Inc.	Medicaid Inc. (2016)	
				Groups with 2-9 EPs			Groups with 10+ EPs							
	Pay Adj. ('18)	PQRS Reporting (Up or neutral Adj) (2016)	+2.0 (x), +1.0 (x), or neutral	Non PQRS Reporting (2018)	PQRS Reporting (Up or Neutral Adj.) (2016)	PQRS Reports (Up or Down Adj.) (2018)	Non PQRS Reporting (2018)	PQRS Reporting (Up or Neutral Adj.) (2016)	PQRS Reporting (Down Adj.) (2018)	Non PQRS Reporting (2018)				

Practitioners

PAs	-2.7% if MIPS	+2.0 (x), +1.0(x), or neutral	2% of MPFS	+2.0 (x), +1.0(x), or neutral	1% net 2% of MPFS	2% of MPFS	+4.0 (x), +2.0(x), or neutral	2% or 4% of MPFS	1% of MPFS	N/A	$8,500 or $21,250	N/A	-2% or -6% of MPFS
NPs													
CNSs													
CRNAs													

	PQRS	Value Modifier	EHR Incentive Program			Total Medicare Payment Adjustments at Risk for Non-Participation in PQRS and Meaningful Use in 2018
	Pay Adj (2018)	Groups and Solo Practitioners	Medicare Inc.	Medicaid Inc. (2016)	Medicare Pay Adj (2018)	

Practitioners

Certified Nurse Midwife	-2.0% of MPFS	N/A	N/A	$8,500 or $21,250 (based on when EP did AIU) / N/A	N/A	-2.0% of MPFS
Clinical Social Worker						
Clinical Psychologist						
Registered Dietician						
Nutrition Professional						
Audiologist						

Therapists

Physical Therapist	-2.0% of MPFS	N/A	N/A	N/A	N/A	-2.0% of MPFS
Occupational Therapist						
Qualified Speech-Language Therapist						

Module 3: 2016 PQRS Updates

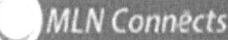

2016 PQRS Updates

- In 2016, 281 measures in the PQRS measure set and 18 measures in the GPRO Web Interface; 23 cross-cutting measures

- Added 3 new measures groups: Multiple Chronic Conditions; Cardiovascular Prevention (Million Hearts); and Diabetic Retinopathy

- Adding the Qualified Clinical Data Registry (QCDR) reporting option for groups in 2016

- 2018 PQRS payment adjustment is the last adjustment that will be issued under PQRS
  - Starting in 2019, adjustments to payment for quality reporting will be made under the Merit-Based Incentive Payment System (MIPS)

2016 PQRS: Reporting Via Claims

- Requirement is to report 9 measures covering at least 3 National Quality Strategy (NQS) domains
  1. Patient Safety
  2. Person and Caregiver-Centered Experience and Outcomes
  3. Communication and Care Coordination
  4. Effective Clinical Care
  5. Community/Population Health
  6. Efficiency and Cost Reduction

- Required to report one "cross-cutting" measure if at least one Medicare face-to-face encounter

- Measure-applicability validation (MAV) process will be used to determine if EP could have reported 9 measures covering at least 3 domains

Individual Reporting Criteria for the 2018 PQRS Payment Adjustment

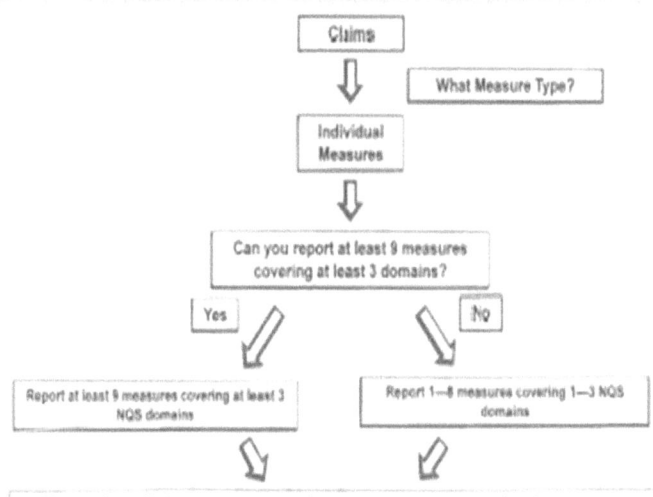

2016 PQRS Cross-Cutting Measures

NQS Domain	Measure Title	Claims	CSV	Registry	EHR	GPRO Web Interface	Measures Group
Community/Population Health	Tobacco Use and Help with Quitting Among Adolescents			X			X
Effective Clinical Care	Hepatitis C: One-Time Screening for Hepatitis C Virus (HCV) for Patients at Risk			X			
Communication and Care Coordination	Medication Reconciliation Post Discharge	X	X				
Communication and Care Coordination	Care Plan	X	X				X
Community/Population Health	Preventive Care and Screening: Influenza Immunization	X	X	<	X		X
Community/Population Health	Pneumonia Vaccination Status for Older Adults	X	X	<	X		X
Effective Clinical Care	Diabetes: Hemoglobin A1c Poor Control	X	X	<	X		X

2016 PQRS Cross-Cutting Measures

NQS Domain	Measure Title	Claims	CSV	Registry	EHR	Large Web Interface	Measures Group
Community/Population Health	Preventive Care and Screening: Body Mass Index (BMI) Screening and Follow-Up Plan	X	X	X	X		X
Patient Safety	Documentation of Current Medications in the Medical Record	X	X	x	X		X
Communication and Care Coordination	Pain Assessment and Follow-Up	X	X				X
Community/Population Health	Preventive Care and Screening: Screening for Clinical Depression and Follow-Up Plan	X	X	X	X		X
Communication and Care Coordination	Functional Outcome Assessment	X	X				
Community/Population Health	Preventive Care and Screening: Tobacco Use: Screening and Cessation Intervention	X	X	X	X		X

APPENDIX # 3
Minimal Data Set 3.0 forms

ASSESSMENTS BASED ON INTERVIEW: GIVING RESIDENTS VOICE

These items contribute to, but do not replace, day-to-day interactions.

Testing has included consideration of "simpler" yes/no formats for these items. If the item asks about something that isn't fixed or absolute, then having more than two response choices can **make responding easier** for older adults. Many adults who struggle with reducing their experience to yes/no will have a much easier time when allowed to select from a range of choices that reflect the variations they actually experience day to day. The response choices have been carefully selected and tested to allow this choice while matching the responses to the question being asked. Both make the task of responding easier.

Some might worry that these type of items dictate to residents and staff about the content of their interactions. Users of structured interviews such as these consistently report that the opposite occurs. Structured questions often bring up important issues for the resident and **open up discussion** between the resident and provider. They help create an ongoing dialogue between the resident and provider within which it is safe to truly report on symptoms and care needs.

Thus, these interview items convey our respect for the resident as a care participant, open important clinical conversations with our residents, increase the accuracy of our assessments, improve the quality of the care we provide and bring nursing home care inline with care in other settings. Most of us talk to our residents every day. We believe that we touch on these important topics and provide ample opportunity for residents to express what they feel. These items ensure that we use part of those conversations to effectively and reliably screen for these important preferences and conditions.

IMPROVEMENTS IN ACCURACY

MDS 3.0 includes changes that seek to improve the accuracy of assessments. For many sections and items, we have included items identified by content experts and research as more valid measures of the condition. Items have been revised based on experience of users and input from subject matter experts who are familiar with nursing home residents and nursing home care. In addition, MDS 3.0 includes modified response options or instructions that aim to increase clarity and therefore agreement across assessors. For example, some items combine response categories where differentiation had been difficult in the past. Instructions for diagnoses have been revised to include detailed algorithms in order to assist in defining active disease. Whenever possible, we have included items or language used in other health care settings in order to improve communication across settings and providers. For example, items included in the National Pressure Ulcer Advisory Panel's PUSH tool are used to describe pressure ulcers; new ADL items separate toilet transfer from toileting and upper body dressing from lower body dressing. The new delirium section is a set of items that have been validated for frail older adults in hospital settings and is based on observations made during structured cognitive assessment. Language has been revised to reflect the standards applied in other settings.

IMPROVEMENTS IN EFFICIENCY

Many of the changes outlined above will increase the efficiency of completing the MDS by yielding higher quality information for the time invested. MDS 3.0 includes other changes that will also increase efficiency. The questions aim for greater consistency in look back windows and test a shorter look back than was used in prior versions. To the extent possible, items that did not address screening for clinical symptoms and syndromes were eliminated. We have, however, retained items that currently form the basis for payment and quality measurement.

Section A — Select Demographic Items

A1. Assessment Reference Date (last day of MDS observation period)

```
__ __  /  __ __  /  __ __ __ __
M  M      D  D       Y  Y  Y  Y
```

A2. Gender

Enter [ ] Code

1. **Male**
2. **Female**

A3. Language

Enter [ ] Code

Does the resident need or want an interpreter to communicate with a doctor or health care staff?

0. **No**
1. **Yes** → If yes, specify primary language: _____
9. **Unable to determine**

A4. Ethnicity

↓ **Complete only on admission assessment** ↓

Enter [ ] Code

Is the resident of Hispanic or Latino origin or descent?

0. **No**
1. **Yes**
9. **Unable to determine**

A5. Race

↓ **Complete only on admission assessment** ↓

Check all that apply.

[ ] a. **American Indian or Alaska Native**
[ ] b. **Asian**
[ ] c. **Black or African American**
[ ] d. **Native Hawaiian or Other Pacific Islander**
[ ] e. **White**
[ ] f. **Other**
[ ] g. **Unable to determine**

A6. Mental Health History

↓ **Complete only on admission assessment** ↓

Enter [ ] Code

The resident has been evaluated by Level II PASRR, and determined to have a serious mental illness and/or mental retardation.

0. **No**
1. **Yes**
9. **Not applicable** (Unit not Medicaid certified)

Section B — Hearing, Speech, and Vision

B1. Comatose

Enter	**Persistent vegetative state/no discernible consciousness** last 5 days.
☐	0. **No**
Code	1. **Yes** ➜ If yes, skip to section G, Functional Status.

B2. Hearing

Enter	**Ability to hear** (with hearing aid or hearing appliance if normally used) last 5 days.
☐	0. **Adequate**—no difficulty in normal conversation, social interaction, listening to TV
Code	1. **Minimal difficulty**—difficulty in some environments (e.g. when person speaks softly or setting is noisy)
	2. **Moderate difficulty**—speaker has to increase volume and speak distinctly
	3. **Highly impaired**—absence of useful hearing

B3. Hearing Aid

Enter	**Hearing aid or other hearing appliance used in above 5-day assessment.**
☐	0. **No**
Code	1. **Yes**

B4. Speech Clarity

Enter	**Select best description of speech pattern in last 5 days.**
☐	0. **Clear speech**—distinct intelligible words
Code	1. **Unclear speech**—slurred, mumbled words
	2. **No speech**—absence of spoken word

B5. Makes Self Understood

Enter	**Ability to express ideas and wants,** consider both verbal and non-verbal expression in last 5 days.
☐	0. **Understood**—clear comprehension
Code	1. **Usually understood**—difficulty communicating some words or finishing thoughts **but** if given time or some prompting is able
	2. **Sometimes understood**—ability is limited to making concrete requests
	3. **Rarely/never understood**

B6. Ability to Understand Others

Enter	**Understanding verbal content,** however able (with hearing aid or device if used) in last 5 days.
☐	0. **Understands**—clear comprehension
Code	1. **Usually understands**—misses some part/intent of message BUT comprehends most conversation
	2. **Sometime understands**—responds adequately to simple, direct communication only
	3. **Rarely/never understands**

B7. Vision

Enter	**Ability to see in adequate light** (with glasses or other visual appliances) in last 5 days.
☐	0. **Adequate**—sees fine detail, including regular print in newspapers/books
Code	1. **Impaired**—sees large print, but not regular print in newspapers/books
	2. **Moderately impaired**—limited vision; not able to see newspaper headlines but can identify objects
	3. **Highly impaired**—object identification in question, but eyes appear to follow objects
	4. **Severely impaired**—no vision or sees only light, colors or shapes; eyes do not appear to follow object

B8. Corrective Lenses

Enter	**Corrective lenses (contacts, glasses, or magnifying glass) used in above 5-day assessment.**
☐	0. **No**
Code	1. **Yes**

Cognitive Patterns

Brief Interview for Mental Status (BIMS)

C1. Interview Attempted

Enter	
☐	
Code	

0. **No** (resident is rarely/never understood or needed interpreter not present) ➜ Skip to C8, Staff Assessment for Mental Status
1. **Yes**

C2. Repetition of Three Words

Enter	
☐	
Code	

Ask resident: "*I am going to say three words for you to remember. Please repeat the words after I have said all three. The words are: sock, blue, and bed. Now tell me the three words.*"

Number of words repeated after first attempt
0. **None**
1. **One**
2. **Two**
3. **Three**

After the resident's first attempt, repeat the words using cues ("sock, something to wear; blue, a color; bed, a piece of furniture"). You may repeat the words up to two more times.

C3. Temporal Orientation (orientation to year, month, and day)

Enter	
☐	
Code	

Ask resident: "*Please tell me what year it is right now.*"

a. **Able to report correct year**
3. **Correct**
2. **Missed by 1 year**
1. **Missed by 2–5 years**
0. **Missed by > 5 years or** no answer

Enter	
☐	
Code	

Ask resident: "*What month are we in right now?*"

b. **Able to report correct month**
2. **Accurate within 5 days**
1. **Missed by 6 days to 1 month**
0. **Missed by >1 month or** no answer

Enter	
☐	
Code	

Ask resident: "*What day of the week is today?*"

c. **Able to report correct day of the week**
1. **Correct**
0. **Incorrect or** no answer

C4. Recall

Ask resident: "*Let's go back to the first question. What were those three words that I asked you to repeat?*" If unable to remember a word, give cue (something to wear; a color; a piece of furniture) for that word.

Enter	
☐	
Code	

a. **Able to recall "sock"**
2. **Yes, no cue required**
1. **Yes, after cueing** ("something to wear")
0. **No**—could not recall

Enter	
☐	
Code	

b. **Able to recall "blue"**
2. **Yes, no cue required**
1. **Yes, after cueing** ("a color")
0. **No**—could not recall

Enter	
☐	
Code	

c. **Able to recall "bed"**
2. **Yes, no cue required**
1. **Yes, after cueing** ("a piece of furniture")
0. **No**—could not recall

C5. Summary Score

Enter Numbers	
☐ ☐	

Add scores for questions C2–C4 and fill in total score (00–15).
Enter 99 if unable to complete interview

C6. Organized Thinking

Enter	
☐	
Code	

a. Ask resident: "*Are there fish in the ocean?*"
1. **Correct** ("yes")
0. **Incorrect or** no answer

Enter	
☐	
Code	

b. Ask resident: "*Does one pound weigh more than two pounds?*"
1. **Correct** ("no")
0. **Incorrect or** no answer

Enter	
☐	
Code	

c. Ask resident: "*Can a hammer be used to pound a nail?*"
1. **Correct** ("yes")
0. **Incorrect or** no answer

C7. Skip Item: Interview Completed

Enter	
☐	
Code	

0. **No** (resident was unable to complete interview) ➜ Continue to C8, Staff Assessment for Mental Status
1. **Yes** ➜ Skip to C12, Signs and Symptoms of Delirium

Cognitive Patterns

Staff Assessment for Mental Status—Complete only if resident interview (C2–C6) not completed

C8. Short Term Memory OK

Enter		Seems or appears to recall after 5 minutes.
	0.	**Memory OK**
Code	1.	**Memory problem**

C9. Long Term Memory OK

Enter		Seems or appears to recall long past.
	0.	**Memory OK**
Code	1.	**Memory problem**

C10. Memory/Recall Ability

Check all that the resident was normally able to recall during the last 5 days:

- ☐ a. **Current season**
- ☐ b. **Location of own room**
- ☐ c. **Staff names and faces**
- ☐ d. **That he or she is in a nursing home**
- ☐ e. **None of the above** is recalled

C11. Cognitive Skills for Daily Decision Making

Enter		Makes decisions regarding tasks of daily life.
	0.	**Independent**—decisions consistent/reasonable
Code	1.	**Modified independent**—some difficulty in new situations only
	2.	**Moderately impaired**—decisions poor; cues/supervision required
	3.	**Severely impaired**—never/rarely made decisions

Delirium

C12. Signs and Symptoms of Delirium (from CAM)

After interviewing the resident, code the following behaviors (a–d) in last 5 days.

Coding:

0. **Behavior not present**

1. **Behavior continuously present, does not fluctuate**

2. **Behavior present, fluctuates** (comes and goes, changes in severity)

→ Enter Codes in Boxes →

a. **Inattention**—Did the resident have difficulty focusing attention (easily distracted, out of touch or difficulty keeping track of what was said)?

b. **Disorganized thinking**—Was the resident's thinking disorganized or incoherent (rambling or irrelevant conversation, unclear or illogical flow of ideas, or unpredictable switching from subject to subject)?

c. **Altered level of consciousness**—Did the resident have altered level of consciousness? (e.g., **vigilant**—startles easily to any sound or touch; **lethargic**—repeatedly dozes off when being asked questions, but responds to voice or touch; **stuporous**—very difficult to arouse and keep aroused for the interview; **comatose**—cannot be aroused)

d. **Psychomotor retardation**—Did the resident have an unusually decreased level of activity such as sluggishness, staring into space, staying in one position, moving very slowly?

C13. Acute Onset Mental Status Change

Enter		Is there evidence of an acute change in mental status from the resident's baseline in last 5 days?
	1.	**Yes**
Code	0.	**No**

Self-Rated Mood Interview—Complete D1–D4 for all residents who are capable of any communication (B5 = 0, 1, or 2), and for whom an interpreter is present or not required.

D1. Interview Attempted

Enter ☐ Code

    0. **No** (resident is rarely/never understood or needed interpreter not present) ➔ Skip to D6, Staff Assessment
    1. **Yes**

D2. Interview (From PHQ-9)

Say to resident: *"Over the last 2 weeks, have you been bothered by any of the following problems?"*	**I. Symptom Presence** If yes, obtain frequency.	**II. Symptom Frequency** Circle one response			
		0. **0–1** **day** (Not at all)	**1.** **2–6** **days** (Several days)	**2.** **7–11** **days** (More than half the days)	**3.** **12–14** **days** (Nearly every day)
a. *Little interest or pleasure in doing things*	Enter ☐ Code 0. **No** 1. **Yes** ➔ 9. **No response**	0	1	2	3
b. *Feeling down, depressed, or hopeless*	Enter ☐ Code 0. **No** 1. **Yes** ➔ 9. **No response**	0	1	2	3
c. *Trouble falling or staying asleep, or sleeping too much*	Enter ☐ Code 0. **No** 1. **Yes** ➔ 9. **No response**	0	1	2	3
d. *Feeling tired or having little energy*	Enter ☐ Code 0. **No** 1. **Yes** ➔ 9. **No response**	0	1	2	3
e. *Poor appetite or overeating*	Enter ☐ Code 0. **No** 1. **Yes** ➔ 9. **No response**	0	1	2	3
f. *Feeling bad about yourself—or that you are a failure or have let yourself or your family down*	Enter ☐ Code 0. **No** 1. **Yes** ➔ 9. **No response**	0	1	2	3
g. *Trouble concentrating on things, such as reading the newspaper or watching television*	Enter ☐ Code 0. **No** 1. **Yes** ➔ 9. **No response**	0	1	2	3
h. *Moving or speaking so slowly that other people could have noticed. Or the opposite-being so fidgety or restless that you have been moving around a lot more than usual*	Enter ☐ Code 0. **No** 1. **Yes** ➔ 9. **No response**	0	1	2	3
i. *Thoughts that you would be better off dead, or of hurting yourself in some way* 1) If i = "Yes", **check here** to indicate that the charge nurse has been informed: ☐	Enter ☐ Code 0. **No** 1. **Yes** ➔ 9. **No response**	0	1	2	3

D3. Total Severity Score

☐☐ Enter Numbers

Sum of all circled frequency responses (D2–II; items a–i). Score may be between 00 and 27. Enter 99 if unable to complete interview (3 or more items in column I marked "No response")
    ☐ **Check here** if some or all frequency responses (D2–II; items a–i) are missing from total score.

D4. Evidence of Depression

Enter | Code
□

Are 2 or more frequency items in <u>shaded</u> columns circled (D2–II, a–i), **and at least one of these is question a or b?**

0. **No**
1. **Yes**

D5. Skip Item: Resident Interview Completed

Enter | Code
□

0. **No** (3 or more items in D2–I, items a–i marked "No response") ➔ Continue to D6, Staff Assessment of Depression
1. **Yes** ➔ Skip to Section E, Behavior

Staff Assessment of Mood—Complete D6–D8 only if resident interview (D1–D5) not completed. (From PHQ-9)

D6. Staff Assessment

		I. Symptom Presence If yes, obtain frequency.	**II. Symptom Frequency** Circle one response			
Say to staff: "Over the last 2 weeks, did the resident have any of the following problems?"			**0.** **0–1** **day** (Not at all)	**1.** **2–6** **days** (Several days)	**2.** **7–11** **days** (More than half the days)	**3.** **12–14** **days** (Nearly every day)
a.	*Little interest or pleasure in doing things*	Enter □ Code 0. **No** 1. **Yes** ➔ 9. **No response**	0	1	2	3
b.	*Feeling down, depressed, or hopeless*	Enter □ Code 0. **No** 1. **Yes** ➔ 9. **No response**	0	1	2	3
c.	*Trouble falling or staying asleep, or sleeping too much*	Enter □ Code 0. **No** 1. **Yes** ➔ 9. **No response**	0	1	2	3
d.	*Feeling tired or having little energy*	Enter □ Code 0. **No** 1. **Yes** ➔ 9. **No response**	0	1	2	3
e.	*Poor appetite or overeating*	Enter □ Code 0. **No** 1. **Yes** ➔ 9. **No response**	0	1	2	3
f.	*Feeling bad about themselves—or that he or she is a failure or has let themselves or their family down*	Enter □ Code 0. **No** 1. **Yes** ➔ 9. **No response**	0	1	2	3
g.	*Trouble concentrating on things, such as reading the newspaper or watching television*	Enter □ Code 0. **No** 1. **Yes** ➔ 9. **No response**	0	1	2	3
h.	*Moving or speaking so slowly that other people could have noticed. Or the opposite- being so fidgety or restless that you have been moving around a lot more than usual*	Enter □ Code 0. **No** 1. **Yes** ➔ 9. **No response**	0	1	2	3
i.	*Thoughts that they would be better off dead, or of hurting themselves in some way* 1) If i = "Yes", **check here** to indicate that the charge nurse has been informed: □	Enter □ Code 0. **No** 1. **Yes** ➔ 9. **No response**	0	1	2	3
j.	*Feeling short-tempered, easily annoyed*	Enter □ Code 0. **No** 1. **Yes** ➔ 9. **No response**	0	1	2	3

Section	Mood
D	

D7. Total Severity Score

Enter Numbers	**Sum of all circled frequency responses** (D6–II, a–i; do not include D6j). Score may be between 00 and 27.
	☐ **Check here** if staff responses are based on observation for less than 14 days.

D8. Evidence of Depression

Enter ☐ Code	**Are 2 or more frequency items in shaded columns circled (D6–II, a–i), and at least one of these is question a or b?** 0. **No** 1. **Yes**

Behavior

E1. Psychosis

Check if problem condition was present at any time in last 5 days:

- [ ] **a.** **Hallucinations** (perceptual experiences in the *absence* of real external sensory stimuli) **or Illusions** (misperceptions in the *presence* of real external sensory stimuli)
- [ ] **b.** **Delusions** (misconceptions or beliefs that are firmly held, contrary to reality)
- [ ] **c.** **None of the above**

Behavioral Symptoms

E2. Behavioral Symptom—Presence & Frequency

Note presence of symptoms and their frequency in the last 5 days:

Coding:
0. **Not present** in last 5 days
1. **Present 1–2 days**
2. **Present 3 or more days**

→ Enter Codes in Boxes [Enter Code]

a. **Physical behavioral symptoms directed toward others** (e.g., hitting, kicking, pushing, scratching, grabbing, abusing others sexually)

[Enter Code]

b. **Verbal behavioral symptoms directed toward others** (e.g., threatening, screaming at others; cursing at others)

[Enter Code]

c. **Other behavioral symptoms not directed toward others** (e.g., physical symptoms such as the resident hitting or scratching Self, pacing, rummaging, public sexual acts, disrobing in public, and throwing or smearing food or bodily wastes, or verbal/vocal symptoms like screaming, disruptive sounds)

→

E3. Overall Presence of Behavioral Symptoms in the last 5 days

[Enter Code]

Were any behavioral symptoms in questions E2 coded 1 or 2?
  0. **No** → Skip to E6, Rejection of Care
  1. **Yes** → Considering all of the symptoms together, answer E4 and E5 below

E4. Impact on Resident

Did any of the identified symptom(s):

[Enter Code]

a. **Put the resident at significant risk for physical illness or injury?**
  0. **No**
  1. **Yes**

[Enter Code]

b. **Significantly interfere with the resident's care?**
  0. **No**
  1. **Yes**

[Enter Code]

c. **Significantly interfere with the resident's participation in activities or social interactions?**
  0. **No**
  1. **Yes**

E5.	**Impact on Others**	

Did any of the identified symptom(s):

Enter ☐ Code	a.	**Put others at clinically significant risk for physical injury?** 0. **No** 1. **Yes**
Enter ☐ Code	b.	**Significantly intrude on the privacy or activity of others?** 0. **No** 1. **Yes**
Enter ☐ Code	c.	**Significantly disrupt care or living environment?** 0. **No** 1. **Yes**

E6.	**Rejection of Care—Presence**	
Enter ☐ Code		In the last 5 days, **did the resident reject evaluation or care** (e.g., bloodwork, taking medications, ADL assistance) **that is necessary to achieve the resident's goals for health and well-being?** Do not include behaviors that have already been addressed (e.g., by discussion or care planning with the resident or family), and/or determined to be consistent with resident values, preferences, or goals. 0. **No** ➜ Skip to E8, Wandering 1. **Yes**

E7.	**Rejection of Care—Frequency**	
Enter ☐ Code		**Number of days on which care was rejected** 1. **1–2 days** 2. **3 or more days**

Wandering

E8.	**Wandering—Presence**	
Enter ☐ Code		In the last 5 days, **has the resident wandered** on at least one occasion? 0. **No** ➜ Skip to E11, Change in Behavioral Symptoms 1. **Yes**

E9.	**Wandering—Impact**	
Enter ☐ Code	a.	**Does the wandering place the resident at significant risk of getting to a place having greater risk of danger** (e.g., stairs, outside of the facility)? 0. **No** 1. **Yes**
Enter ☐ Code	b.	**Does the wandering significantly intrude on the privacy or activities of others?** 0. **No** 1. **Yes**

E10. Wandering—Frequency		
Enter ☐ Code		**Of the last 5 days, on how many days has wandering occurred?** 1. **1–2 days** 2. **3 or more days**

E11.	**Change in Behavioral or Other Symptoms**—Consider all of the symptoms assessed in items E1 through E10.
⬇	**Complete only on follow-up assessment** ⬇
Enter ☐ Code	How does resident's current behavior status, care rejection, or wandering **compare to last assessment?** 0. **Same** 1. **Improved** 2. **Worse**

F1.   Preferred Routine

<u>All</u> residents should be asked about preferences. Complete F1 for all residents who are capable of any communication (B5 is coded 0, 1, or 2), and for whom an interpreter is present or not required. For residents who are not able to communicate, interview family member, or significant other who knows the resident and can provide information on past customs and preferences.

Preface a–h by saying to resident: *"While you are in the nursing home…"*

Coding:		
	Enter [Code]	**a.** How important is it to you to **choose what clothes to wear?**
	Enter [Code]	**b.** How important is it to you to **take care of your personal belongings or things?**
→	Enter [Code]	**c.** How important is it to you to **choose between a tub bath, shower, bed bath, or sponge bath?**
	Enter [Code]	**d.** How important is it to you to have **snacks available between meals?**
	Enter [Code]	**e.** If you could go to bed whenever you wanted, how important would it be to you to **stay up past 8:00 p.m.?**
→	Enter [Code]	**f.** How important is it to you to have your **family or a close friend involved in discussions about your care?**
	Enter [Code]	**g.** How important is it to you to be able to **use the phone in private?**
	Enter [Code]	**h.** How important is it to you to have a **place to lock your things** to keep them safe?

Coding:
1. *Very important*
2. *Somewhat important*
3. *Not very important*
4. *Not important at all*
5. *Important, but can't do or no choice*
9. *No response or non-responsive*

Enter Codes in Boxes

F2.   Primary Respondent

Enter [Code]   Indicate primary respondent for F1, Preferred Routine:

1. **Resident**
2. **Significant Other** (family, close friend, or other representative)
9. **Could not be completed by resident or significant other**

Preferences for Customary Routine, Activities, Community Setting

F3. Activity Pursuit Patterns

<u>All</u> residents who are able to communicate should be asked about activity pursuit patterns—even if they have not been able to complete F1. Complete F3 for all residents who are capable of any communication (B5 is coded 0, 1, or 2), and for whom an interpreter is present or not required. For residents who are not able to communicate, interview family, or significant other who knows the resident and can provide information on past customs and preferences.

Preface a–j by saying to resident: *"While you are in the nursing home…"*

Coding: 1. *Very important* 2. *Somewhat important* 3. *Not very important* 4. *Not important at all* 5. *Important, but can't do or no choice* 9. *No response or non-responsive*	➔ **Enter Codes in Boxes** ➔	**Enter** ☐ **Code** **a.** How important is it to you to have **books, newspapers, and magazines** to read?
		Enter ☐ **Code** **b.** How important is it to you to listen to **music** you like?
		Enter ☐ **Code** **c.** How important is it to you to be around **animals** such as pets?
		Enter ☐ **Code** **d.** How important is it to you to keep up with the **news**?
		Enter ☐ **Code** **e.** How important is it to you to do things with **groups of people**?
		Enter ☐ **Code** **f.** How important is it to you to do your **favorite activities**?
		Enter ☐ **Code** **g.** How important is it to you to do things **away from the nursing home**?
		Enter ☐ **Code** **h.** How important is it to you to **go outside** to get fresh air when the weather is good?
		Enter ☐ **Code** **i.** How important is it to you to participate in **religious services or practices**?

Enter ☐ **Code** **j.** If your doctor approves, would you like to be offered **alcohol on occasion** at meals or social events?
   0. *No*
   1. *Yes*
   5. *Yes, but can't do or no choice*
   9. *No response or non-responsive answer*

F4. Primary Respondent

Enter ☐ **Code** Indicate primary respondent for F3, Activity Pursuit Patterns:
   1. **Resident**
   2. **Significant Other** (family, close friend, or other representative)
   9. **Could not be completed by resident or significant other**

F5. **Return to Community**

⬇ **Complete only on admission assessment** ⬇

Ask resident (or family or significant other if resident unable to respond):

Enter		
☐	*"Do you want to talk to someone about the possibility of **returning to the community?"***	
Code	0. **No**	
	1. **Yes**	

F6. **Skip Item: Staff Assessment Required**

Enter	Was either F2, Preferred Routine Respondent, or F4, Activity Respondent coded 9?
☐	0. **No** ➔ Skip to Section G, Functional Status
Code	1. **Yes** ➔ Complete F7, Staff Assessment of Activity and Daily Preferences

---

F7. **Staff Assessment of Activity and Daily Preferences**—Complete only if unable to interview resident or other representative for either F1, Preferred Routine, or F3, Activity Pursuit Patterns.

Resident Prefers:

☐	a.	Choosing clothes to wear	☐	k.	Place to lock personal belongings
☐	b.	Caring for personal belongings	☐	l.	Reading books, newspapers, or magazines
☐	c.	Receiving tub bath	☐	m.	Listening to music
☐	d.	Receiving shower	☐	n.	Being around animals such as pets
☐	e.	Receiving bed bath	☐	o.	Keeping up with the news
☐	f.	Receiving sponge bath	☐	p.	Doing things with groups of people
☐	g.	Snacks between meals	☐	q.	Participating in favorite activities
☐	h.	Staying up past 8:00 p.m.	☐	r.	Spending time away from the nursing home
☐	i.	Family or close friend involvement in care discussions	☐	s.	Spending time outdoors
			☐	t.	Participating in religious activities or practices
☐	j.	Use of phone in private	☐	u.	None of the above

Check all that apply (left and right columns)

Functional Status

G1. Activities of Daily Living (ADL) Assistance

Code for most dependent episode in last 5 days:

Coding:

0. **Independent**—resident completes activity with no help or oversight

1. **Set up assistance**

2. **Supervision**—oversight, encouragement or cueing provided throughout the activity

3. **Limited assistance**—guided maneuvering of limbs or other non-weight bearing assistance provided at least once

4. **Extensive assistance, 1 person assist**— resident performed part of the activity while one staff member provided weight-bearing support or completed part of the activity at least once →

5. **Extensive assistance, 2 + person assist**— resident performed part of the activity while two or more staff members provided weight-bearing support or completed part of the activity at least once

6. **Total dependence, 1 person assist**—full staff performance of activity (requiring only 1 person assistance) at least once. The resident must be unable or unwilling to perform any part of the activity. →

7. **Total dependence, 2 + person assist**—full staff performance of activity (requiring 2 or more person assistance) at least once. The resident must be unable or unwilling to perform any part of the activity.

8. **Activity did not occur** during entire period

Enter Codes in Boxes

Enter ▭ Code **a.** **Bed mobility** moving to and from lying position, turning side to side and positioning body while in bed.

Enter ▭ Code **b.** **Transfer** moving between surfaces—to or from: bed, chair, wheelchair, standing position (**excludes** to/from bath/toilet).

Enter ▭ Code **c.** **Toilet transfer** how resident gets to and moves on and off toilet or commode.

Enter ▭ Code **d.** **Toileting** using the toilet room (or commode, bedpan, urinal); cleaning self after toileting or incontinent episode(s), changing pad, managing ostomy or catheter, adjusting clothes (**excludes** toilet transfer).

Enter ▭ Code **e.** **Walk in room** walking between locations in his/her room.

Enter ▭ Code **f.** **Walk in facility** walking in corridor or other places in facility.

Enter ▭ Code **g.** **Locomotion** moving about facility, with wheelchair if used.

Enter ▭ Code **h.** **Dressing upper body** dressing and undressing above the waist, includes prostheses, orthotics, fasteners, pullovers.

Enter ▭ Code **i.** **Dressing lower body** dressing and undressing from the waist down, includes prostheses, orthotics, fasteners, pullovers.

Enter ▭ Code **j.** **Eating** includes eating, drinking (regardless of skill) or intake of nourishment by other means (e.g., tube feeding, total parenteral nutrition, IV fluids for hydration).

Enter ▭ Code **k.** **Grooming/personal hygiene** includes combing hair, brushing teeth, shaving, applying makeup, washing/drying face and hands (**excludes** bath and shower).

Enter ▭ Code **l.** **Bathing** how resident takes full-body bath/shower, sponge bath and transfers in/out of tub/shower (**excludes** washing of back and hair).

G2. **Mobility Prior to Admission**

↓ Complete only on admission assessment ↓

Enter	a.	Did resident have a **hip fracture, hip replacement, or knee replacement** in the 30 days prior to this admission?

☐ Code

        0. **No** ➔ Skip to G3, Balance During Transitions and Walking

        1. **Yes** ➔ Complete G2b

        9. **Unable to determine** ➔ Skip to G3, Balance During Transitions and Walking

b. **If yes, check all that apply for tasks in which the resident was independent prior to fracture/replacement.**

☐   1. **Transfer**

☐   2. **Walk across room**

☐   3. **Walk 1 block on a level surface**

☐   4. **Resident was not independent in any of these activities**

☐   9. **Unable to determine**

G3. **Balance During Transitions and Walking**

After observing the resident, code the following **walking and transition items for most dependent** over the last 5 days:

Coding:

0. **Steady at all times**

1. Not steady, but __able__ to stabilize without human assistance

2. Not steady, __only able__ to stabilize with human assistance

3. **Activity did not occur**

→ Enter Codes in Boxes →

Enter ☐ Code	a.	**Moving from seated to standing** position
Enter ☐ Code	b.	**Walking** (with assistive device if used)
Enter ☐ Code	c.	**Turning around** and facing the opposite direction while walking
Enter ☐ Code	d.	**Moving on and off toilet**
Enter ☐ Code	e.	**Surface-to-surface transfer** (transfer from wheelchair to bed or bed to wheelchair)

G4. **Functional limitation in range of motion**

Code for limitation during last 5 days that interfered with daily functions or placed resident at risk of injury.

Coding:

0. **No impairment**

1. **Impairment on one side**

2. **Impairment on both sides**

→ Enter Codes in Boxes →

Enter ☐ Code	a.	**Lower extremity** (hip, knee, ankle, foot)
Enter ☐ Code	b.	**Upper extremity** (shoulder, elbow, wrist, hand)

Functional Status

G5. Gait and Locomotion

Check all that were normally used in the past 5 days:

- ☐ a. **Cane/Crutch**
- ☐ b. **Walker**
- ☐ c. **Wheelchair (manual or electric)**
- ☐ d. **Limb prosthesis**
- ☐ e. **None of the above** were used

G6. Bedfast

Enter ☐ Code

In bed or in recliner in room for more than 22 hours on at least three of the past 5 days.

    0. **No**
    1. **Yes**

G7. Functional Rehabilitation Potential

↓   **Complete only on admission assessment**   ↓

Enter ☐ Code

a.   **Resident believes s/he is capable of increased independence** in at least some ADL's.

    0. **No**
    1. **Yes**
    9. **Unable to determine**

Enter ☐ Code

b.   **Direct care staff believe resident is capable of increased independence** in at least some ADL's.

    0. **No**
    1. **Yes**

Bladder and Bowel

H1. Urinary Appliances

Check all that applied in last 5 days:

- [ ] a. **Indwelling bladder catheter**
- [ ] b. **External (condom) catheter**
- [ ] c. **Ostomy (suprapubic catheter, ileostomy)**
- [ ] d. **Intermittent catheterization**
- [ ] e. **None of the above**

H2. Urinary Continence

Enter
Code

Urinary continence in last 5 days. Select the one category that best describes the resident over the last 5 days:
- 0. **Always continent**
- 1. **Occasionally incontinent** (less than 5 episodes of incontinence)
- 2. **Frequently incontinent** (5 or more episodes of incontinence but at least one episode of continent voiding)
- 3. **Always incontinent** (no episodes of continent voiding)
- 9. **Not rated**, resident had a catheter (indwelling, condom), urinary ostomy, or no urine output for entire 5 days

H3. Urinary Incontinence Management

Enter
Code

a. **Has a trial of a toileting program (e.g. scheduled toileting, prompted voiding, or bladder training) been attempted** on admission or since urinary incontinence was noted in this facility?
- 0. **No** → Skip to item H4, Bowel Continence
- 1. **Yes**
- 9. **Unable to determine**

Enter
Code

b. **Response**—What was the resident's response to the trial program?
- 0. **No improvement**
- 1. **Decreased wetness**
- 2. **Completely dry** (continent)
- 9. **Unable to determine**

Enter
Code

c. **Current toileting program**—Is a toileting program currently being used to manage the resident's urinary incontinence?
- 0. **No**
- 1. **Yes**

H4. Bowel Continence

Enter
Code

Bowel continence in last 5 days. Select the one category that best describes the resident over the last 5 days:
- 0. **Always continent**
- 1. **Occasionally incontinent** (one episode of bowel incontinence)
- 2. **Frequently incontinent** (2 or more episodes of bowel incontinence but at least one continent bowel movement)
- 3. **Always incontinent** (no episodes of continent bowel movements)
- 9. **Not rated,** resident had an ostomy or did not have a bowel movement for the entire 5 days

H5. Bowel Patterns

Enter
Code

Constipation present in the past 5 days?
- 0. **No**
- 1. **Yes**

Active Disease Diagnosis

Active Diseases in the last 30 days

Cancer

☐ 1. **Cancer** (with or without metastasis)

Heart/Circulation

☐ 2. **Anemia** (includes aplastic, iron deficiency, pernicious, and sickle cell)

☐ 3. **Atrial Fibrillation and Other Dysrhythmias** (includes bradycardias, tachycardias)

☐ 4. **Coronary Artery Disease** (includes angina, myocardial infarction)

☐ 5. **Deep Venous Thrombosis/ Pulmonary Embolus**

☐ 6. **Heart Failure** (includes pulmonary edema)

☐ 7. **Hypertension**

☐ 8. **Peripheral Vascular Disease/Peripheral Arterial Disease**

☐ 9. **Other Heart/ Circulation:** enter diagnosis and ICD-9:_____

Gastrointestinal

☐ 10. **Cirrhosis**

☐ 11. **GERD/Ulcer** (includes esophageal, gastric, and peptic ulcers)

☐ 12. **Ulcerative Colitis/ Chrohn's Disease/Inflammatory Bowel Disease**

☐ 13. **Other Gastrointestinal:** enter diagnosis and ICD-9:_____

Genitourinary

☐ 14. **Benign Prostatic Hyperplasia**

☐ 15. **Renal Insufficiency**

☐ 16. **Other Genitourinary:** enter diagnosis and ICD-9:_____

Infections

☐ 17. **Human Immunodeficiency Virus (HIV) Infection** (includes AIDS)

☐ 18. **MRSA, VRE, Clostridium diff. Infection / Colonization**

☐ 19. **Pneumonia**

☐ 20. **Tuberculosis**

☐ 21. **Urinary Tract Infection**

☐ 22. **Viral Hepatitis** (includes Hepatitis A, B, C, D, and E)

☐ 23. **Wound Infection**

☐ 24. **Other Infections:** enter diagnosis and ICD-9:_____

Metabolic

☐ 25. **Diabetes Mellitus** (includes diabetic retinopathy, nephropathy, and neuropathy)

☐ 26. **Hyponatremia**

☐ 27. **Hyperkalemia**

☐ 28. **Hyerlipidemia**

☐ 29. **Thyroid Disorder** (Includes hypothyroidism, hyperthyroidism, and Hashimoto's thyroiditis)

☐ 30. **Other Metabolic:** enter diagnosis and ICD-9:_____

Musculoskeletal

☐ 31. **Arthritis** (Degenerative Joint Disease, Osteoarthritis, and Rheumatoid Arthritis)

☐ 32. **Osteoporosis**

☐ 33. **Hip Fracture** (includes any hip fracture that continues to have a relationship to current status, treatments, monitoring. Includes sub-capital fractures, fractures of the trochanter and femoral neck) (last 90 days)

☐ 34. **Other Fracture**

☐ 35. **Other Musculoskeletal:** enter diagnosis and ICD-9:_____

Neurological

☐ 36. **Alzheimer's Disease**

☐ 37. **Aphasia**

☐ 38. **Cerebral Palsy**

☐ 39. **CVA/ TIA/ Stroke**

☐ 40. **Dementia** (Non-Alzheimer's dementia, including vascular or multi-infarct dementia, mixed dementia, frontotemporal dementia (e.g., Pick's disease), and dementia related to stroke, Parkinson's, Huntington's, Pick's, or Creutzfeldt-Jakob diseases)

☐ 41. **Hemiplegia/Hemiparesis/Paraplegia/Quadriplegia**

☐ 42. **Multiple Sclerosis**

☐ 43. **Parkinson's Disease**

☐ 44. **Seizure Disorder**

☐ 45. **Traumatic Brain Injury**

☐ 46. **Other Neurological:** enter diagnosis and ICD-9:_____

Nutritional

☐ 47. **Protein Calorie Malnutrition** or at risk for malnutrition

☐ 48. **Other Nutritional:** enter diagnosis and ICD-9:_____

Psychiatric/Mood Disorder

☐ 49 **Anxiety Disorder**

☐ 50. **Depression** (other than Bipolar)

☐ 51. **Manic Depression** (Bipolar Disease)

☐ 52. **Schizophrenia**

☐ 53. **Other Psychiatric/Mood Disorder:** enter diagnosis and ICD-9:_____

Pulmonary

☐ 54. **Asthma/ COPD Chronic Lung Disease** (includes restrictive lung diseases such as asbestosis and chronic bronchitis)

☐ 55. **Other Pulmonary:** enter diagnosis and ICD-9:_____

Other

☐ 56. **Note Additional Diagnoses:** enter diagnosis and ICD-9:_____

ICD-9:_____

ICD-9:_____

ICD-9:_____

ICD-9:_____

Check all that apply.

J1.	**Pain Management** (answer for all residents, regardless of current pain level)	
	At any time in the last 5 days, has the resident:	
Enter ☐ Code	a.	**Been on a scheduled pain medication regimen?** 0. **No** 1. **Yes**
Enter ☐ Code	b.	**Received PRN pain medications?** 0. **No** 1. **Yes**
Enter ☐ Code	c.	**Received non-medication intervention for pain?** 0. **No** 1. **Yes**

Pain Assessment Interview—<u>All</u> residents should be asked about pain. Complete J2–J7 for all residents who are capable of any communication (B5 is coded 0, 1, or 2), and for whom an interpreter is present or not required.

J2.	**Interview Attempted**	
Enter ☐ Code		0. **No** (resident is rarely/never understood or needed interpreter is not present) ➜ Skip to J9, Staff Assessment of Pain 1. **Yes**
J3.	**Pain Presence**	
Enter ☐ Code		Ask resident: *"**Have you had pain or hurting** at any time in the last 5 days?"* 0. **No** ➜ Skip to J8, Interview Completed 1. **Yes** ➜ Proceed to items J4–J8 below 9. **Unable to answer** ➜ Skip to J8, Interview Completed
J4.	**Pain Frequency**	
Enter ☐ Code		Ask resident: *"**How much of the time** have you experienced pain or hurting over the last 5 days?"* 1. *Almost constantly* 2. *Frequently* 3. *Occasionally* 4. *Rarely* 9. **Unable to answer**
J5.	**Pain Effect on Function**	
Enter ☐ Code	a.	Ask resident: *"Over the past 5 days, **has pain made it hard for you to sleep at night?**"* 0. **No** 1. **Yes** 9. **Unable to answer**
Enter ☐ Code	b.	Ask resident: *"Over the past 5 days, **have you limited your day-to-day activities because of pain?**"* 0. **No** 1. **Yes** 9. **Unable to answer**

Health Conditions

J6.	Pain Intensity—Administer **one** of the following pain intensity questions (a or b)

a. **Verbal Descriptor Scale**
Ask resident: *"Please rate the intensity of your worst pain over the last 5 days"*
(Show resident verbal scale.)
1. *Mild*
2. *Moderate*
3. *Severe*
4. *Very severe, horrible*
9. **Unable to answer** or **not attempted**

Enter Code

b. **Numeric Rating Scale (00–10)**
Ask resident:
"Please rate your worst pain over the last 5 days on a zero to ten scale with zero being no pain and ten as the worst pain you can imagine."
(Show resident 0–10 pain scale.)
Enter two-digit response. Enter 99 if unable to answer or **not attempted.**

Enter Number

c. **Indicate which Pain Intensity question was administered.**
1. **Verbal Descriptor Scale only**
2. **Numeric Rating Scale (00–10) only**
3. **Both were tried and one scale completed**
9. **Both were tried, and neither scale completed**

Enter Code

J7.	**Pain Treatment Goals**

Ask resident: *"In your opinion, how important is it for your pain treatment to* **completely eliminate** *your pain?"*
1. *Extremely important*
2. *Very important*
3. *Somewhat important*
4. *Not at all important*
9. **Unable to answer**

Enter Code

J8.	**Skip Item: Interview Completed**

0. **No** (Resident was unable to answer whether pain was present in J3, **or** unable to answer 3 or more pain descriptors in items J4–J7) ➜ Proceed to J9, Staff Assessment for Pain
1. **Yes** ➜ Skip to J10, Shortness of Breath

Enter Code

Staff Assessment for Pain

J9.	**Staff Assessment for Pain**—Complete only if pain interview (J2–J8) not completed

Indicators of pain or possible pain in the last 5 days. Check all that apply:

- a. **Non-verbal sounds** (crying, whining, gasping, moaning, or groaning)
- b. **Vocal complaints of pain** (that hurts, ouch, stop)
- c. **Facial expressions** (grimaces, winces, wrinkled forehead, furrowed brow, clenched teeth or jaw)
- d. **Protective body movements or postures** (bracing, guarding, rubbing or massaging a body part/area, clutching or holding a body part during movement)
- e. **None of these signs observed or documented**

Other Health Conditions

J10. Shortness of Breath (dypsnea)

Select all that apply in last 5 days:

- ☐ a. **Shortness of breath or trouble breathing with exertion** (e.g. walking, bathing, transferring)
- ☐ b. **Shortness of breath or trouble breathing when sitting at rest**
- ☐ c. **Shortness of breath or trouble breathing when lying flat**
- ☐ d. **None of the above**

J11. Cough Present

Enter | **Cough present** in last 5 days.
☐ | 0. **No**
Code | 1. **Yes**

J12. Chest Pain or Angina

Select all that apply in last 5 days:

- ☐ a. **Chest pain or angina with exertion** (e.g. walking, bathing, transferring)
- ☐ b. **Chest pain or angina when sitting or at rest**
- ☐ c. **None of the above**

J13. Current Tobacco Use

Enter | **Tobacco use** in last 5 days.
☐ | 0. **No**
Code | 1. **Yes**

J14. Prognosis

Enter | Does the resident have a condition or chronic disease that may result in a **life expectancy of less than 6 months**?
☐ | Requires physician documentation. If not documented, discuss with physician and request supporting documentation)
Code | 0. **No**
| 1. **Yes**

Falls Assessment

J15. Skip Item for Falls: Admission or Follow-up

Enter Code	What assessment type are you completing?
	1. **Admission assessment** → Complete J16, Fall History (Admission)
	2. **Follow-up assessment (quarterly or annual)** → Skip to J17, Any Falls Since Last Assessment

J16. Fall History (Admission)

↓ **Complete J16a-d only on Admission Assessment** ↓

Enter Code	a.	Did the resident fall one or more times in the **30 days** (i.e., month) before admission?
		0. **No**
		1. **Yes**
		9. **Unable to determine**
Enter Code	b.	Did the resident fall one or more times in the **31–180 days** (i.e., 1–6 months) before admission?
		0. **No**
		1. **Yes**
		9. **Unable to determine**
Enter Code	c.	Did the resident have any **fracture related to a fall in the 6 months** prior to admission?
		0. **No**
		1. **Yes**
		9. **Unable to determine**
Enter Code	d.	Has the resident **fallen since admission** to the nursing home?
		0. **No** → Skip to Section K, Swallowing
		1. **Yes** → Skip to Section K, Swallowing

J17. Any Falls Since Last Assessment (Quarterly or Annual Assessment)

↓ **Complete J17 only on Quarterly or Annual Assessment** ↓

Enter Code	Has the resident **had any falls since the last assessment?**
	0. **No** → Skip to Section K, Swallowing
	1. **Yes**

J18. Number of Falls Since Last Assessment (Quarterly or Annual Assessment)

↓ **Complete only on Quarterly or Annual Assessment** ↓

Code the number of falls in each category since the last assessment.

	Enter Codes in Boxes			
Coding: 0. **None** 1. **One** 2. **Two or more**	→	Enter Code	a.	**No injury**—no evidence of any injury is noted on physical assessment by the nurse or primary care clinician; no complaints of pain or injury by the resident; no change in the resident's behavior is noted after the fall
	→	Enter Code	b.	**Injury (except major)**—skin tears, abrasions, lacerations, superficial bruises, hematomas and sprains; or any fall-related injury that causes the resident to complain of pain
	→	Enter Code	c.	**Major injury**—bone fractures, joint dislocations, closed head injuries with altered consciousness, subdural hematoma

Section K Swallowing/Nutritional Status

K1. Swallowing Disorder

Signs and symptoms of possible swallowing disorder. Check all that applied in last 5 days:

☐	a.	Loss of liquids/solids from mouth when eating or drinking
☐	b.	Holding food in mouth/cheeks or residual food in mouth after meals
☐	c.	Coughing or choking during meals or when swallowing medications
☐	d.	Complaints of difficulty or pain with swallowing
☐	e.	None of the above

K2. Height and Weight

☐☐ inches	a.	**Height** (in inches) most recent height measure since admission. (If height includes a fraction, round up to nearest inch.)
☐☐☐ pounds	b.	**Weight** (in pounds) base weight on most recent measure in last 30 days; measure weight consistently, according to standard facility practice (e.g., in a.m. after voiding, before meal, with shoes off, etc.) (If weight includes a fraction, round up to nearest pound.)

K3. Weight Loss

Enter ☐ Code	**Loss of 5% or more in last 30 days** (or since last assessment if sooner) **or loss of 10% or more in last 180 days.** 0. **No** or unknown 1. **Yes**, planned loss 2. **Yes**, unplanned loss

K4. Nutritional Approaches

Check all that applied in last 5 days:

☐	a.	**Parenteral/IV feeding**
☐	b.	**Feeding-tube**—nasogastric or abdominal (PEG)
☐	c.	**Mechanically altered diet**—require change in texture of food or liquids (e.g., pureed food, thickened liquids)
☐	d.	**Therapeutic diet** (low salt, diabetic, low cholesterol)
☐	e.	**None of the above**

K5. Percent Intake by Artificial Route ➔ Skip to Section L, Oral/Dental Status, if neither K4a or K4b is checked

Enter ☐ Code	a.	**Proportion of total calories the resident received through parenteral or tube feedings** in the last 5 days. 1. **25% or less** 2. **26–50%** 3. **51% or more**
Enter ☐ Code	b.	**Average fluid intake per day by IV or tube** in last 5 days. 1. **500 cc/day or less** 2. **501 cc/day or more**

Section L — Oral/Dental Status

L1. Dental

Check all that applied in last 5 days:

Check all that apply

- ☐ **a.** **Broken or loosely fitting denture or partial** (chipped, cracked, uncleanable, or loose)
- ☐ **b.** **No natural teeth or tooth fragment(s)** (edentulous)
- ☐ **c.** **Abnormal mouth tissue** (ulcers, masses, oral lesions, including under denture or partial if one is worn)
- ☐ **d.** **Obvious cavity or broken natural teeth**
- ☐ **e.** **Inflamed or bleeding gums or loose natural teeth**
- ☐ **f.** **Mouth or facial pain,** discomfort or difficulty with chewing
- ☐ **g.** **None of the above** were present
- ☐ **h.** **Unable to examine**

Skin Conditions

M1. Current Pressure Ulcer

Enter	**Did the resident have a pressure ulcer in the last 5 days?**
☐ Code	0. **No** → Skip to M11, Healed Pressure Ulcers, Page 26
	1. **Yes**

M2. Stage 1 Ulcers

Report based on highest stage of existing ulcer(s) at its worst; do not reverse stage.

Enter ☐ Number	**Number of existing pressure ulcers at Stage 1**—Observable pressure-related alteration of an area of intact skin whose indicators may include change in: skin temperature (warm or cool), tissue consistency (firm or boggy feel), or sensation (pain, itching). In lightly pigmented skin, appears as an area of persistent redness. In darker skin tones, may appear with persistent red, blue, or purple hues.

M3. Stage 2 Ulcers

Report based on highest stage of existing ulcer(s) at its worst; do not reverse stage.

Enter ☐ Number	a.	**Number of existing pressure ulcers at Stage 2**—Partial thickness skin loss involving epidermis, dermis, or both. The ulcer presents clinically as an abrasion, blister, or shallow crater. **If number entered = 0 → Skip to M4, Stage 3 ulcers.**
Enter ☐ Number	b.	**Number of these Stage 2 pressure ulcers that were present on admission.** Of the pressure ulcers listed in M3a, how many were first noted at Stage 2 within 48 hours of admission and not acquired in the facility?
Length (cm) ☐☐.☐ Width (cm) ☐☐.☐	c.	**Current dimensions of largest Stage 2 pressure ulcer.** Enter 99.9 if unable to determine (for study purposes only).

M4. Stage 3 Ulcers

Report based on highest stage of existing ulcer(s) at its worst; do not reverse stage.

Enter ☐ Number	a.	**Number of existing pressure ulcers at Stage 3**—Full thickness skin loss involving damage to, or necrosis of, subcutaneous tissue that may extend down to, but not through, underlying fascia. The ulcer presents clinically as a deep crater with or without undermining of adjacent tissue. **If number entered = 0 → Skip to M5, Stage 4 ulcers.**
Enter ☐ Number	b.	**Number of these Stage 3 pressure ulcers that were present on admission.** Of the pressure ulcers listed in M4a, how many were first noted at Stage 3 within 48 hours of admission and not acquired in the facility?
Length (cm) ☐☐.☐ Width (cm) ☐☐.☐ Depth (cm) ☐☐.☐	c.	**Current dimensions of largest Stage 3 pressure ulcer.** Enter 99.9 if unable to determine (for study purposes only).

M5. Stage 4 Ulcers

Report based on highest stage of existing ulcer(s) at its worst; do not reverse stage.

Enter ☐ Number	a.	**Number of existing pressure ulcers at Stage 4**—Full thickness skin loss with extensive destruction, tissue necrosis, or damage to muscle, bone, or supporting structures (e.g., tendon, joint, capsule). Undermining and sinus tracts also may be associated with Stage 4 pressure ulcers. **If number entered = 0 → Skip to M6, Nonstageable ulcers.**
Enter ☐ Number	b.	**Number of these Stage 4 pressure ulcers that were present on admission.** Of the pressure ulcers listed in M5a, how many were first noted at Stage 4 within 48 hours of admission and not acquired in the facility?
Length (cm) ☐☐.☐ Width (cm) ☐☐.☐ Depth (cm) ☐☐.☐	c.	**Current dimensions of largest Stage 4 pressure ulcer.** Enter 99.9 if unable to determine (for study purposes only).

M6. Nonstageable Ulcers

Enter ▢ Number
a. **Not Stageable**—Cannot be observed due to presence of eschar that is intact and fully adherent to edges of wound or wound covered with non-removable dressing/cast and no prior staging known.

Enter ▢ Number
b. **Number of these nonstageable pressure ulcers that were present on admission.** Of the pressure ulcers listed in M6a, how many were first noted as nonstageable within 48 hours of admission and not acquired in the facility?

M7. Exudate Amount for Most Advanced Stage

Enter ▢ Code
Select the item that best describes the **amount of exudate in the largest pressure ulcer at the most advanced stage.**

0. **None**
1. **Light**
2. **Moderate**
3. **Heavy**
9. **Not observable/not documented**

M8. Tissue Type for Most Advanced Stage

Enter ▢ Code
Select the item that best describes the **type of tissue present in the ulcer bed of the largest pressure ulcer at the most advanced stage.**

0. **Closed/resurfaced**—completely covered with epithelium
1. **Epithelial Tissue** —new skin growing in superficial ulcer
2. **Granulation Tissue** —pink or red tissue with shiny, moist, granular appearance
3. **Slough**—yellow or white tissue that adheres to the ulcer bed in strings or thick clumps, or is mucinous
4. **Necrotic Tissue (Eschar)** —black, brown, or tan tissue that adheres firmly to the wound bed or ulcer edges, may be softer or harder than surrounding skin.
9. **Not observable/not documented**

M9. Data Source for Current Pressure Ulcer items (M2–M8)

This item is for study analysis purposes; not for consideration for MDS 3.0.

Enter ▢ Code
Select the data source used for information on pressure ulcers.

1. **Research nurse direct observation with facility nurse**
2. **Facility nurse completing MDS 3.0 assessment**
3. **Chart review**

M10. Worsening in Pressure Ulcer Status Since Last Assessment

Indicate the number of current pressure ulcers that were **not present or were at a lesser stage** on last MDS (if no current pressure ulcer at a given stage, enter 0).

▢ a. **Check here if N/A** (no prior assessment)

Enter ▢ Number
b. **Stage 2**

Enter ▢ Number
c. **Stage 3**

Enter ▢ Number
d. **Stage 4**

Section M Skin Conditions

M11. Healed Pressure Ulcers

Indicate the number of pressure ulcers that were noted on last MDS that have **completely healed.** (If no current pressure ulcer at a given stage, enter 0).

☐ a. **Check here if N/A** (no prior assessment **or** no pressure ulcers on prior assessment)

Enter [ ] Number b. **Stage 2**

Enter [ ] Number c. **Stage 3**

Enter [ ] Number d. **Stage 4**

M12. Other Ulcers, Wounds, and Skin Problems

Check all that apply in the past 5 days:

☐ a. **Venous or arterial ulcer(s)**
☐ b. **Diabetic foot ulcer(s)**
☐ c. **Other foot or lower extremity infection** (cellulitis)
☐ d. **Surgical wound(s)**
☐ e. **Open lesion(s) other than ulcers, rashes, cuts** (e.g., cancer lesion)
☐ f. **Burn(s)**
☐ g. **None of the above** were present

M13. Skin Treatments

Check all that apply in the past 5 days:

☐ a. **Pressure reducing device for chair**
☐ b. **Pressure reducing device for bed**
☐ c. **Turning/repositioning program**
☐ d. **Nutrition or hydration intervention** to manage skin problems
☐ e. **Ulcer care**
☐ f. **Surgical wound care**
☐ g. **Application of dressings** (with or without topical medications) other than to feet
☐ h. **Applications of ointments/medications** other than to feet
☐ i. **None of the above** were provided

Section N	**Medications**

N1. Injections

[ ] Days — Record the **number of days that injectable medications were received** during the last 5 days or since admission if less than 5 days.

N2. Medications Received

Check all medications the resident received at any time during the last 5 days or since admission if less than 5 days:

Check all that apply

- [ ] a. **Antipsychotic**
- [ ] b. **Antianxiety**
- [ ] c. **Antidepressant**
- [ ] d. **Hypnotic**
- [ ] e. **Anticoagulant** (warfarin, heparin, or low-molecular weight heparin)
- [ ] f. **None of the above**

Special Treatments and Procedures

O1. Special Treatments and Programs

	↓ Complete for all Assessments ↓ **I.** Past 5 days, **or** since admission if less than 5 days	↓ Complete only for ↓ **5-day Assessment** **II.** In 5 days prior to admission
		Check here if not a 5-day assessment: ☐
Cancer Treatment		➔ Skip this column
a. **Chemotherapy**	☐	☐
b. **Radiation**	☐	☐
Respiratory Treatments		
c. **Oxygen therapy**	☐	☐
d. **Suctioning**	☐	☐
e. **Tracheostomy care**	☐	☐
f. **Ventilator or respirator**	☐	☐
Other		
g. **IV medications**	☐	☐
h. **Transfusions**	☐	☐
i. **Dialysis**	☐	☐
j. **Hospice care**	☐	☐
k. **Respite care**	☐	☐
l. **Isolation or quarantine** for active infectious disease (does not include standard body/fluid precautions)	☐	☐
m. **None of the above**	☐	☐

Check all that apply.

O2. Influenza Vaccine

Enter ___ Code

a. Did the **resident receive the Influenza Vaccine in this facility** for this year's Influenza season (October 1 through March 31)?

    0. **No**
    1. **Yes** ➔ Skip to O3, Pneumococcal Vaccine
    9. **Does not apply because assessment outside influenza season** ➔ Skip to O3, Pneumococcal Vaccine

Enter ___ Code

b. If **Influenza Vaccine not received, state reason:**

    1. **Not in facility** during this year's flu season
    2. **Received outside of this facility**
    3. **Not eligible**
    4. **Offered and declined**
    5. **Not offered**
    6. **Inability to obtain vaccine** due to declared shortage
    7. **None of the above**

O3. Pneumococcal Vaccine

Enter ___ Code

a. Is the resident's **Pneumococcal Vaccine status up to date?**

    0. **No**
    1. **Yes** ➔ Skip to O4, Therapies

Enter ___ Code

b. If **Pneumococcal Vaccine not received, state reason:**

    1 **Not eligible**
    2. **Offered and declined**
    3. **Not offered**
    4. **Vaccine status not up to date by admission ARD**

Special Treatments and Procedures

O4. Therapies

Record the **number of days each of the following therapies was administered** for at least 15 minutes a day in the last 5 calendar days (column I). Enter 0 if none or less than 15 minutes daily. For Therapies a–c also record the total number of minutes (column II). Note: Count only post admission therapies.

I. Days	II. Minutes				
☐	☐ ☐ ☐	**a.**	Speech-language pathology and audiology services		
☐	☐ ☐ ☐	**b.**	Occupational Therapy		
☐	☐ ☐ ☐	**c.**	Physical Therapy		
☐		**d.**	Respiratory Therapy		
☐		**e.**	Psychological Therapy (by any licensed mental health professional)		
☐		**f.**	Recreational Therapy (includes recreational and music therapy)		

O5. Nursing Rehabilitation/ Restorative Care

Record the **number of days** each of the following rehabilitative or restorative techniques was administered (for at least 15 minutes a day) in the last 5 calendar days (enter 0 if none or less than 15 minutes daily).

Number of Days		
☐	**a.**	**Range of motion (passive)**
☐	**b.**	**Range of motion (active)**
☐	**c.**	**Splint or brace assistance**
		Training and skill practice in:
☐	**d.**	**Bed mobility**
☐	**e.**	**Transfer**
☐	**f.**	**Walking**
☐	**g.**	**Dressing or grooming**
☐	**h.**	**Eating or swallowing**
☐	**i.**	**Amputation/prostheses care**
☐	**j.**	**Communication**

O6. Physician Examinations

☐ Days	Over the last 5 days, **on how many days did the physician (or authorized assistant or practitioner) examine the resident?**

O7. Physician Orders

☐ Days	Over the last 5 days, **on how many days did the physician (or authorized assistant or practitioner) change the resident's orders?**

Section P | Restraints

P1. Physical Restraints

Physical restraints are any manual method, physical or mechanical device, material or equipment attached or adjacent to the resident's body that the individual cannot remove easily, which restricts freedom of movement or normal access to one's body. Code for last 5 days:

		Used in Bed
	Enter [ ] Code	a. Full bed rails on all open sides of the bed
	Enter [ ] Code	b. Other type of side rail used (e.g., half rail, one side)
	Enter [ ] Code	c. Trunk restraint
Coding: **0. Not used** **1. Used less than daily** **2. Used daily**	→ Enter [ ] Code	d. Limb restraint
	Enter [ ] Code	e. Other
		Used in Chair or Out of Bed
	→ Enter [ ] Code	f. Trunk restraint
	Enter [ ] Code	g. Limb restraint
	Enter [ ] Code	h. Chair prevents rising
	Enter [ ] Code	i. Other

(Column label: Enter Codes in Boxes)

Section Q · Participation in Assessment and Goal Setting

Q1. Participation in Assessment

Enter Code [ ]
a. **Resident**
   0. **No**
   1. **Yes**

Enter Code [ ]
b. **Family**
   0. **No**
   1. **Yes**
   9. **No family**

Enter Code [ ]
c. **Significant other**
   0. **No**
   1. **Yes**
   9. **None**

Q2. Resident's Overall Goals

↓ **Complete only on Admission Assessment** ↓

Enter Code [ ]
a. **Select one for resident's goals established during assessment process.**
   1. **Post acute care**—expects to **return to community**
   2. **Post acute care**—expects to have **continued NH needs**
   3. **Respite stay**—expects to **return home**
   4. **Other reason for admit**—expects to **return to community.**
   5. **Long term care** for medical, functional, and/or cognitive impairments
   6. **End-of-life care**
   9. **Unknown or uncertain**

Enter Code [ ]
b. **Indicate information source for this item**
   1. **Resident**
   2. **Close family member or significant other**
   3. **Neither**

APPENDIX # 4
Senate Subcommittees

"The list of Senate Subcommittees"

Source: The Committee System in the U.S. Congress, Congressional Research Service, Library of Congress. August 29, 1994, revised by the Senate Historical Office, September 2002.

About the Senate Committee System:

Due to the high volume and complexity of its work, the Senate divides its tasks among 20 committees, 68 subcommittees, and 4 joint committees. Although the Senate committee system is similar to that of the House of Representatives, it has its own guidelines, within which each committee adopts its own rules. This creates considerable variation among the panels.

Standing committees generally have legislative jurisdiction. Subcommittees handle specific areas of the committee's work. Select and joint committees generally handle oversight or housekeeping responsibilities.

The chair of each committee and a majority of its members represent the majority party. The chair primarily controls a committee's business. Each party assigns its own members to committees, and each committee distributes its members among its subcommittees. The Senate places limits on the number and types of panels any one senator may serve on and chair.

Committees receive varying levels of operating funds and employ varying numbers of aides. Each hires its own staff. The majority party controls most committee staff and resources, but a portion is shared with the minority.

Several thousand bills and resolutions are referred to committees during each 2-year Congress. Committees select a small percentage for consideration, and those not addressed often receive no further action. The bills that committees report help to set the Senate's agenda.

When a committee or subcommittee favors a measure, it usually takes four actions. First it asks relevant executive agencies for written comments on the measure. Second, it holds hearings to gather information and views from non-committee experts. At committee hearings, these witnesses summarize submitted statements and then respond to questions from the senators. Third, a committee meets to perfect the measure through amendments, and non-committee members sometimes attempt to influence the language. Fourth, when language is agreed upon, the committee sends the measure back to the full Senate, usually along with a written report describing its purposes and provisions.

A committee's influence extends to its enactment of bills into law. A committee that considers a measure will manage the full Senate's deliberation on it. Also, its members will be appointed to any conference committee created to reconcile its version of a bill with the version passed by the House of Representatives.

Other types of committees deal with the confirmation or rejection of presidential nominees. Committee hearings that focus on the implementation and investigation of programs are known as oversight hearings, whereas committee investigations examine allegations of wrongdoing.

About House Committees:

The House's 20 standing committees have different legislative jurisdictions. Each considers bills and issues and recommends measures for consideration by the House. Committees also have oversight responsibilities to monitor agencies, programs, and activities within their jurisdictions, and in some cases in areas that cut across committee jurisdictions.

Current standing committees of the House: Agriculture; Appropriations; Armed Services; Budget; Commerce; Education and the Workforce; Ethics; Financial Services; Foreign Affairs; Homeland Security; House Administration; Judiciary; Natural Resources; Oversight and Government Reform; Rules; Science, Space, and Technology; Small Business; Transportation and Infrastructure; Veterans' Affairs; and Ways and Means.

The Committee of the Whole House is a committee of the House on which all representatives serve and which meets in the House Chamber for the consideration of measures from the Union calendar.

Before members are assigned to committees, each committee's size and the proportion of Republicans to Democrats must be decided by the party leaders. The total number of committee slots allotted to each party is approximately the same as the ratio between majority party and minority party members in the full chamber.

Additional information as to the specific committees and congressmen assigned just google the subcommittees and more information is available to all.

APPENDIX # 5
Comprehensive Primary Care

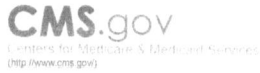

(http://www.cms.gov)

Innovation Center Home (/index.html) ➤ Innovation Models (/initiatives/index.html) ➤ Comprehensive Primary Care Plus

Comprehensive Primary Care Plus

Share

Comprehensive Primary Care Plus (CPC+) is a national advanced primary care medical home model that aims to strengthen primary care through a regionally-based multi-payer payment reform and care delivery transformation. CPC+ will include two primary care practice tracks with incrementally advanced care delivery requirements and payment options to meet the diverse needs of primary care practices in the United States (U.S.). The care delivery redesign ensures practices in each track have the infrastructure to deliver better care to result in a healthier patient population. The multi-payer payment redesign will give practices greater financial resources and flexibility to make appropriate investments to improve the quality and efficiency of care, and reduce unnecessary health care utilization. CPC+ will provide practices with a robust learning system, as well as actionable patient-level cost and utilization data feedback, to guide their decision making.

CPC+ is a five-year model that will begin in January 2017.

Background

Strengthening primary care is critical to promoting health and reducing overall health care costs in the U.S. CPC+ builds on the foundation of the Comprehensive Primary Care (CPC) initiative, a model tested through the Center for Medicare & Medicaid Innovation that runs from October 2012 through December 31, 2016. CPC+ integrates many lessons learned from CPC, including insights on practice readiness, the progression of care delivery redesign, actionable performance-based incentives, necessary health information technology, and claims data sharing with practices.

CPC+ will bring together CMS, commercial insurance plans, and State Medicaid agencies to provide the financial support necessary for practices to make fundamental changes in their care delivery. CMS will enter into a Memorandum of Understanding (MOU) with selected payer partners to document a shared commitment to align on payment, data sharing, and quality metrics throughout the five year initiative.

Model Details

The goal of CPC+ is to improve the quality of care patients receive, improve patients' health, and spend health care dollars more wisely. Practices in both tracks will make changes in the way they deliver care, centered on key Comprehensive Primary Care Functions: (1) Access and Continuity; (2) Care Management; (3) Comprehensiveness and Coordination; (4) Patient and Caregiver Engagement; and (5) Planned Care and Population Health. Additional information about each CPC+ track is listed below:

	Track 1	Track 2
Practice Capabilities	Pathway for practices ready to build the capabilities to deliver comprehensive primary care.	Pathway for practices poised to increase the comprehensiveness of care through enhanced Health IT, improve care of patients with complex needs, and inventory of resources and supports to meet patients' psychosocial needs.
Medicare Care Management Fee	Average Medicare care management fee of $15 per beneficiary per month.	Average Medicare care management fee of $28 per beneficiary per month, which includes a $100 care management fee for patients with the most complex needs.
Medicare Payment Structure	Practices will receive regular fee-for-service payments.	Practices will receive "Comprehensive Primary Care Payments (CPCP)" – a hybrid of Medicare fee-for-service and a percentage of their expected Evaluation & Management (E&M) reimbursements upfront in the form of a CPCP. Practices will receive a commensurate reduction in E&M fee-for-service payments for a percentage of claims.
Medicare Performance-Based Incentive Payment	Practices are eligible for a performance-based incentive payment of $2.50 per beneficiary per month. Incentive payments are prepaid at the beginning of a performance year, but practices may only keep these funds if quality and utilization performance thresholds are met.	Practices are eligible for a performance-based incentive payment of $4 per beneficiary per month. Incentive payments are prepaid at the beginning of a performance year, but practices may only keep these funds if quality and utilization performance thresholds are met.

4/19/2016 11:10 PM

Health IT Vendor Partner	N/A	Practices must submit a letter of support from their health IT vendor(s) that outlines vendors' commitment to supporting practices with advanced health IT capabilities.
Medicare Payment Structure	Practices will receive regular fee-for-service payments.	Practices will receive "Comprehensive Primary Care Payments (CPCP)" – a hybrid of Medicare fee-for-service and a percentage of their expected Evaluation & Management (E&M) reimbursements upfront in the form of a CPCP. Practices will receive a commensurate reduction in E&M fee-for-service payments for a percentage of claims.
Multi-Payer Support	Practices must have support from multiple payers partnering in CPC+.	Payers must have support from multiple payers partnering in CPC+.

How to Apply

Payer solicitation and practice applications will be a staggered process. First, CMS will solicit payer proposals to partner with Medicare in CPC+ (April 15-June 1, 2016). The choice of up to 20 CPC+ regions will be informed by the geographic reach of selected payers.

Next, CMS will publicize the CPC+ regions, and solicit applications from practices within these regions (July 15-September 1, 2016). Practices will apply directly to the track for which they believe they are ready; however, CMS reserves the right to offer practice entrance into Track 1 if they apply to, but do not meet the eligibility requirements for Track 2.

Practices applying to Track 2 will need to submit a letter of support from their Health IT vendor(s) that outlines vendors' commitment to supporting the practice with advanced health IT capabilities. CMS will sign a Memorandum of Understanding with those health IT vendors supporting Track 2 practices selected to participate in CPC+.

Stakeholder Webinars

CMS will host webinars on the following dates for interested stakeholders:

CPC+ Model Announcement – open to all members of the public

Thursday, April 14 | 3:00 – 4:00 p.m. EDT | Registration is open (https://engage.vevent.com/rt/cms2~041416j) (//www.cms.gov/About-CMS/Agency-Information/Aboutwebsite/External-Link-Disclaimer.html)

Tuesday, April 19 | 3:00 – 4:00 p.m. EDT | Registration is open (https://engage.vevent.com/rt/cms2~041916pm) (//www.cms.gov/About-CMS/Agency-Information/Aboutwebsite/External-Link-Disclaimer.html)

CPC+ Health IT Vendor Event – open to Health IT vendors only

Thursday, April 21 | 12:00 – 1:00p.m. EDT | Registration is open (https://cms-cmmi-meetings.webex.com/mw0401lsp13/mywebex/default.do?nomenu=true&siteurl=cms-cmmi-meetings&service=6&rnd=0.5971449757876779&main_url=https%3A%2F%2Fcms-cmmi-meetings.webex.com%2Fec0701lsp13%2Feventcenter%2Fevent%2FeventAction.do%3FtheAction%3Ddetail%26confViewID%3D3571688%26%26EMK%3D4832534b00000002eb0e8188304d1381ac62176f347fda63c3463c38683036b534def106369f8be3%25%26%26siteurl%3Dcms-cmmi-meetings) (//www.cms.gov/About-CMS/Agency-Information/Aboutwebsite/External-Link-Disclaimer.html)

CPC+ Interested Payer Event – open to payers only

Wednesday, April 27 | 2:00 – 3:00p.m. EDT | Registration is open (https://cms-cmmi-meetings.webex.com/mw0401lsp13/mywebex/default.do?nomenu=true&siteurl=cms-cmmi-meetings&service=6&rnd=0.51005946506693144&main_url=https%3A%2F%2Fcms-cmmi-meetings.webex.com%2Fec0701lsp13%2Feventcenter%2Fevent%2FeventAction.do%3FtheAction%3Ddetail%26confViewID%3D3571694%26%26EMK%3D4832534b0000002ada23105e3b24fe924cadf2ebc7861288bc79cd7f71e23318f637305795f1793%25%26%26siteurl%3Dcms-cmmi-meetings) (//www.cms.gov/About-CMS/Agency-Information/Aboutwebsite/External-Link-Disclaimer.html)

Tuesday, May 10 | 2:00 – 3:00p.m. EDT | Registration is open (https://cms-cmmi-meetings.webex.com/mw0401lsp13/mywebex/default.do?nomenu=true&siteurl=cms-cmmi-meetings&service=6&rnd=0.51005946506693144&main_url=https%3A%2F%2Fcms-cmmi-meetings.webex.com%2Fec0701lsp13%2Feventcenter%2Fevent%2FeventAction.do%3FtheAction%3Ddetail%26confViewID%3D3571720%26%26EMK%3D4832534b0000000292bccf5180132a08655f9d9f6a24ab5991576af9b6465be06364091be11e85f%26%26%26siteurl%3Dcms-cmmi-meetings) (//www.cms.gov/About-CMS/Agency-Information/Aboutwebsite/External-Link-Disclaimer.html)

For questions about the model or the solicitation process, please email CPCplus@cms.hhs.gov (mailto:CPCplus@cms.hhs.gov)

Additional Information

CPC+ Request for Applications (PDF) (/Files/x/cpcplus-rfa.pdf)
CPC+ Payer Solicitation (PDF) (/Files/x/cpcplus-payersolicitation.pdf)
CPC+ Payer Memorandum of Understanding (PDF) (/Files/x/cpcplus-payermou.pdf)
CPC+ Press Release (https://www.cms.gov/Newsroom/MediaReleaseDatabase/Press-releases/2016-Press-releases-items/2016-04-11.html)
CPC+ Fact Sheet (https://www.cms.gov/Newsroom/MediaReleaseDatabase/Fact-sheets/2016-Fact-sheets-items/2016-04-11.html)
Frequently Asked Questions (PDF) (/Files/x/cpcplus-faqs.pdf)
JAMA article, "Medicare's Vision for Advanced Primary Care: New Directions for Care Delivery and Payment" (April 11, 2016)
(http://jama.jamanetwork.com/article.aspx?doi=10.1001/jama.2016.4472) or (//www.cms.gov/About-CMS/Agency-Information/Aboutwebsite
/External-Link-Disclaimer.html)

Page Not Found

The page you are looking for could not be found. Please chec

Model Summary

Stage: Announced
Number of Participants: N/A
Category: Primary Care Transformation
Authority: Section 3021 of the Affordable
Care Act

Milestones & Updates

Apr 19, 2016
Announced: Payer memorandum of
understanding (MOU) posted

Apr 11, 2016
Announced: National primary care medical
home model aims to strengthen primary
care through regionally-based multi-payer
transformation

Where Health Care
Innovation is
Happening

(/initiatives/map/index.html)
See who's working with CMS to
implement new payment and
service delivery models.

**Get the Widget
(/CMMIMapWidget
/index.html)**

Related Items

Primary Care Transformation

Advanced Primary Care Initiatives

Stage: Under Development
Learn More (/initiatives/Advanced-
Primary-Care/)

Primary Care Transformation

**Comprehensive Primary Care
Initiative**

Stage: Ongoing
Learn More (/initiatives
/Comprehensive-Primary-
Care-Initiative/)

Primary Care Transformation

Comprehensive Primary Care Plus

Stage: Announced
Learn More (/initiatives
/comprehensive-primary-care-plus/)

Last updated on: 04/19/2016

CMS.gov

A federal government website managed by the Centers for Medicare & Medicaid Services
7500 Security Boulevard, Baltimore, MD 21244

(http://www.hhs.gov)

CMS & HHS Websites

Medicare.gov (http://www.medicare.gov)
MyMedicare.gov (http://MyMedicare.gov)
StopMedicareFraud.gov
(http://www.stopmedicarefraud.gov)
Medicaid.gov (http://Medicaid.gov)
InsureKidsNow.gov
(http://www.insurekidsnow.gov)
HealthCare.gov (http://www.HealthCare.gov)
HHS.gov/Open (http://www.hhs.gov/open/)

Tools

Acronyms (http://www.cms.gov/apps/acronyms)
Contacts (http://www.cms.gov/apps/contacts)
FAQs (https://questions.cms.gov/)
Glossary (http://www.cms.gov/apps/glossary/)
Archive (http://archive-it.org/collections/2744)

Helpful Links

Web Policies & Important Links (http://www.cms.gov/About-CMS/Agency-Information/Aboutwebsite
/index.html)
Privacy Policy (http://www.cms.gov/About-CMS/Agency-Information/Aboutwebsite/Privacy-Policy.html)
Plain Language (http://www.medicare.gov/about-us/plain-writing/plain-writing.html)
Freedom of Information Act (http://www.cms.gov/center/freedom-of-information-act-center.html)
No Fear Act (http://www.cms.gov/About-CMS/Agency-Information/Aboutwebsite/NoFearAct.html)
Nondiscrimination/Accessibility (http://www.cms.gov/About-CMS/Agency-Information/Aboutwebsite
/CMSNondiscriminationNotice.html)
HHS.gov (http://www.hhs.gov)
Inspector General (http://oig.hhs.gov)
USA.gov (http://www.usa.gov)
Help with file formats & plug-ins (http://www.cms.gov/About-CMS/Agency-Information/Aboutwebsite
/Help.html)

Receive Email Updates

APPENDIX # 6

Example of the Federal Register

§71.1 [Amended]

■ 2. The incorporation by reference in 14 CFR 71.1 of FAA Order 7400.9X, Airspace Designations and Reporting Points, dated August 7, 2013 and effective September 15, 2013, is amended as follows:

Paragraph 6010(a) Domestic VOR Federal Airways

*   *   *   *   *

V–44 [Amended]

From Columbia, MO; INT Columbia 131° and Foristell, MO, 262° radials; Foristell; Centralia, IL; to Samsville, IL. From Falmouth, KY; York, KY; Parkersburg, WV; Morgantown, WV; Martinsburg, WV; INT Martinsburg 094° and Baltimore, MD, 300° radials; Baltimore: INT Baltimore 122° and Sea Isle, NJ, 267° radials; Sea Isle; INT Sea Isle 040° and Deer Park, NY, 209° radials; Deer Park; INT Deer Park 041° and Bridgeport, CT, 133° radials; Bridgeport; INT Bridgeport 324° and Pawling, NY, 160° radials; Pawling; INT Pawling 342° and Albany, NY, 181° radials; to Albany. The airspace within R–4001B, R–5002A, R–5002B, and R–5002E is excluded when active. The airspace within V–139 and V–308 airways is excluded. The airspace below 2,000 feet MSL outside the United States is excluded.

*   *   *   *   *

V–47 [Amended]

From Pine Bluff, AR; Gilmore, AR; Dyersburg, TN; Cunningham, KY; to Pocket City, IN. From Cincinnati, OH; Rosewood, OH; Flag City, OH; to Waterville, OH.

*   *   *   *   *

V–49 [Amended]

From Vulcan, AL; Decatur, AL; Nashville, TN; Bowling Green, KY; to Mystic, KY.

*   *   *   *   *

V–51 [Amended]

From Pahokee, FL; INT Pahokee 010°and Treasure, FL, 193° radials; Treasure; INT Treasure 330°and Ormond Beach, FL, 183° radials; Ormond Beach; Craig, FL; Alma, GA; Dublin, GA; Athens, GA; INT Athens 340°and Harris, GA, 148° radials; Harris; Hinch Mountain, TN; Livingston, TN; to Louisville, KY. From Shelbyville, IN; INT Shelbyville 313° and Boiler, IN, 136° radials; Boiler; to Chicago Heights, IL.

*   *   *   *   *

Issued in Washington, DC, on August 7, 2014.

Gary A. Norek,

Manager, Airspace Policy and Regulations Group.

[FR Doc. 2014–19210 Filed 8–14–14; 8:45 am]

BILLING CODE 4910–13–P

DEPARTMENT OF THE TREASURY

Internal Revenue Service

26 CFR Part 1

[TD 9688]

RIN 1545–BJ64

Retail Inventory Method

AGENCY: Internal Revenue Service (IRS), Treasury.

ACTION: Final regulations.

SUMMARY: This document contains final regulations relating to the retail inventory method of accounting. The regulations restate and clarify the computation of ending inventory values under the retail inventory method and provide a special rule for certain taxpayers that receive margin protection payments or vendor allowances that are required to reduce only cost of goods sold. The regulations affect taxpayers that are retailers and use a retail inventory method.

DATES: *Effective Date:* These regulations are effective on August 15, 2014.

Applicability Date: For date of applicability, see § 1.471–8(f).

FOR FURTHER INFORMATION CONTACT: Christopher Call, (202) 317–7007 (not a toll-free number).

SUPPLEMENTARY INFORMATION:

Background

This document contains final regulations that amend the Income Tax Regulations (26 CFR part 1) relating to the retail inventory method of accounting under § 1.471–8 of the Income Tax Regulations. On October 7, 2011, a notice of proposed rulemaking (REG–125949–10) was published in the Federal Register (76 FR 62327). A public hearing was not requested or held. No comments were received during the comment period. Three comments were received after the end of the comment period and were considered, as discussed later in this preamble. The proposed regulations are adopted as amended by this Treasury decision.

Summary of Comments and Explanation of Revisions

Section 471 of the Internal Revenue Code provides that a taxpayer's method of accounting for inventories must clearly reflect income. Section 1.471–2(c) provides that the bases of inventory valuation most commonly used and meeting the requirements of section 471 are (1) cost and (2) cost or market, whichever is lower (LCM). Section 1.471–3 provides rules for determining

inventories at cost. Section 1.471–4 provides rules for determining inventories at lower of cost or market. Section 1.471–8 of the regulations contains rules specific to retailers, allowing them to approximate cost or LCM of the goods in their ending inventory by using the retail inventory method. Under the retail inventory method, a taxpayer computes the value of ending inventory by multiplying a cost complement by the retail selling prices of the goods on hand at the end of the taxable year. The numerator of the cost complement is the value of beginning inventory plus the cost of purchases during the taxable year, and the denominator is the retail selling prices of beginning inventory plus the initial retail selling prices of purchases. For taxpayers using the retail inventory method to value inventories at cost (retail cost method), the denominator of the cost complement is adjusted for all permanent markups and markdowns. Taxpayers using the retail inventory method to value inventories at LCM (retail LCM method) generally do not make adjustments to the denominator for markdowns.

The proposed regulations provided that a taxpayer using the retail LCM method may not reduce the numerator of the cost complement by the amount of an allowance, discount, or price rebate that is related to or intended to compensate for a permanent reduction in the taxpayer's retail selling price of inventory, often called a margin protection payment or a markdown allowance. The proposed regulations also provided that a taxpayer using the retail inventory method (whether valuing inventories at LCM or at cost) may not reduce the numerator of the cost complement by the amount of a sales-based vendor allowance.

Commenters suggested that taxpayers using the retail LCM method to value inventories should reduce the numerator of the cost complement for all vendor allowances and discounts, including margin protection payments and sales-based vendor allowances (but should not be required to reduce the denominator by the related selling price reduction), because all allowances and discounts reduce the cost of inventory and allow retailers to achieve their margin goals. The commenters asserted that if the numerator of the cost complement is not reduced for margin protection payments and sales-based vendor allowances, taxpayers' income will not be clearly reflected, the economics of the underlying business transaction will be ignored, and small retailers would be adversely affected. The commenters suggested that small retailers have less bargaining power than large retailers and are less able to negotiate purchase-based discounts from vendors.

The final regulations do not adopt these comments. A margin protection payment, unlike other types of allowances, is inherently related to a markdown that will be reflected in the retail selling prices of the items remaining in ending inventory. When a taxpayer using retail LCM reduces the numerator of the cost complement by the amount of a margin protection payment without reducing the denominator by the amount of the corresponding markdown, ending inventory value does not clearly reflect income, and does not reflect the economics of the underlying transaction. Taxpayers using the retail cost method to value inventories, as opposed to retail LCM, are allowed to reduce the numerator of the cost complement by the amount of a margin protection payment because these taxpayers also reduce the denominator of the cost complement by the amount of a related markdown, maintaining the relationship between cost and retail price.

With regard to sales-based vendor allowances, the final regulations adopt, with a modification, the proposed rule that the numerator of the cost complement is not reduced for sales-based vendor allowances. Proposed regulations under § 1.471–3(e) provided that sales-based vendor allowances (the amount of an allowance, discount, or price rebate that a taxpayer earns by selling specific merchandise) reduce cost of goods sold and do not reduce ending inventory value. Because the retail inventory method produces an ending inventory value and sales-based vendor allowances could not be allocated to ending inventory, the proposed regulations under § 1.471–8 provided that sales-based vendor allowances do not reduce the numerator of the cost complement. The final regulations under § 1.471–3(e) (TD 9652, 79 FR 2094) apply specifically to only one type of sales-based vendor allowance, a sales-based vendor chargeback, and reserve rules for other types of sales-based vendor allowances. To conform to this modification, these final regulations under § 1.471–8 provide that sales-based vendor allowances that are required to reduce only cost of goods sold under § 1.471–3(e) do not reduce the numerator of the cost complement. This rule will apply only to sales-based vendor chargebacks until further guidance is issued under § 1.471–3(e).

Commenters also requested that the final regulations allow retail LCM taxpayers to reduce the numerator of the cost complement by margin protection payments and sales-based vendor allowances because requiring taxpayers to track margin protection payments and sales-based vendor allowances separately from other types of allowances would create burdensome recordkeeping requirements. This comment is not adopted because, as discussed earlier in this preamble, allowing a retail LCM taxpayer to reduce the numerator of the cost complement by the amount of a margin protection payment without reducing the denominator by the amount of the corresponding markdown would not clearly reflect income and would not reflect the economics of the underlying transaction. Nonetheless, as discussed later in this preamble, to ease taxpayers' compliance burden, the final regulations provide alternative methods and procedures for computing the cost complement for retail LCM taxpayers.

The preamble to the proposed regulations requested comments on an alternative method for retail LCM taxpayers to account for margin protection payments when computing the cost complement. The method described in that preamble would have permitted retail LCM taxpayers to reduce the numerator of the cost complement for all non-sales-based allowances, discounts, or price rebates, including margin protection payments or markdown allowances, and also would have required a reduction of the denominator of the cost complement for permanent markdowns to which the margin protection payments or markdown allowances relate (related markdowns). Although commenters did not address this proposal explicitly, they stated that in some cases, based on the nature of their business dealings with vendors and the variety of allowances offered, taxpayers have difficulty distinguishing between the different types of vendor allowances their vendors provide. For example, commenters contend that it might be difficult for a taxpayer to distinguish the amount of a margin protection payment or markdown allowance received from a vendor from the amounts of other types of allowances received from that vendor, thus making it difficult to determine the amount by which they were required to reduce the numerator of the cost complement under the proposed regulations.

The final regulations address these comments and ease taxpayers' compliance with the regulations by allowing retail LCM taxpayers to use a

method similar to the method described in the preamble to the proposed regulations that does not require taxpayers to distinguish the amounts of margin protection payments from the amounts of other vendor allowances (except for vendor allowances required to be allocated to cost of goods sold under § 1.471–3(e)). Under the alternative method provided in the final regulations, retail LCM taxpayers reduce the numerator for margin protection payments and must quantify and reduce the denominator for the related markdowns. This alternative method results in a reduction of the numerator of the cost complement by all vendor allowances other than those required to reduce cost of goods sold under § 1.471–3(e). This alternative method accordingly reduces the compliance burden for taxpayers that cannot distinguish margin protection payments from other allowances, but that can identify the markdowns related to those margin protection payments.

Commenters also stated that some accounting systems cannot sufficiently track the related markdowns. Accordingly, a second alternative provided in the final regulations allows taxpayers that are able to determine the amount of their margin protection payments to reduce the numerator of the cost complement for the margin protection payments and adjust the denominator by the amount that, in conjunction with the reduction of the numerator, maintains what would have been the cost complement percentage before taking into account the margin protection payments and related markdowns. This second alternative method assumes that a margin protection payment maintains the taxpayer's profit margin after a related markdown in retail selling price. Thus, if before taking into account the margin protection payment and the related markdown the cost complement is 50 percent ($10/$20), and the taxpayer receives a margin protection payment of $2, the taxpayer must reduce the denominator by $4 to maintain a cost complement of 50 percent ($8/$16) under this second alternative method.

A retail LCM taxpayer must use one of these three methods (the general method and the two alternative methods) for computing all of its cost complements. A change from one to another of those methods is a change in method of accounting.

The final regulations further facilitate identifying margin protection payments and related markdowns by allowing retail LCM taxpayers to use statistical sampling in accordance with Rev. Proc. 2011–42 (2011–37 IRB 318), see

§ 601.601(d), in conjunction with any of the three methods. A retail LCM taxpayer using statistical sampling must use it for all margin protection payments and related markdowns associated with the inventory items valued by a particular cost complement. However, a retail LCM taxpayer that calculates more than one cost complement is not required to use statistical sampling for all cost complements. A change from using to not using statistical sampling, or from not using to using statistical sampling, to identify margin protection payments and related markdowns is not a change in method of accounting.

The proposed regulations provided that a taxpayer may apply the retail inventory method to a department, a class of goods, or a stock-keeping unit. A commenter suggested that the final regulations specify that a taxpayer may use the retail inventory method to value ending inventory for a sub-class of goods, style of goods, or other similar category of goods to avoid the implication that the scope of the retail inventory method is limited to those groupings specifically identified in the proposed regulations. The categories suggested by the commenter are already encompassed by the terms department, class of goods, or stock-keeping unit. Accordingly, the final regulations do not adopt this comment.

A commenter suggested that the final regulations should allow taxpayers to calculate their cost complements using a measurement period shorter than the entire taxable year and should clarify whether beginning inventory may or must be eliminated from the cost complement of a last-in, first-out (LIFO) taxpayer using the retail inventory method. These issues were not addressed in the proposed regulations and therefore are not addressed in the final regulations. However, the final regulations do not reflect a change in established administrative practice regarding whether LIFO taxpayers using the retail inventory method may exclude beginning inventory from the cost complement.

Effective/Applicability Date

These regulations apply to taxable years beginning after December 31, 2014. For taxable years beginning before January 1, 2015, see § 1.471–0 as contained in 26 CFR part 1, revised April 1, 2014.

Special Analyses

This Treasury decision is not a significant regulatory action as defined in Executive Order 12866, as supplemented by Executive Order

13563. Therefore, a regulatory assessment is not required. Section 553(b) of the Administrative Procedure Act (5 U.S.C. chapter 5) does not apply to these regulations and, because the regulations do not impose a collection of information on small entities, the Regulatory Flexibility Act (5 U.S.C. chapter 6) does not apply. Pursuant to section 7805(f) of the Internal Revenue Code, the notice of proposed rulemaking that preceded these final regulations was submitted to the Chief Counsel for Advocacy of the Small Business Administration for comment on its impact on small business. No comments were received from the Small Business Administration.

Drafting Information

The principal author of these regulations is Natasha M. Mulleneaux of the Office of Associate Chief Counsel (Income Tax and Accounting). However, other personnel from the IRS and the Treasury Department participated in their development.

List of Subjects in 26 CFR Part 1

Income taxes, Reporting and recordkeeping requirements.

Adoption of Amendments to the Regulations

Accordingly, 26 CFR part 1 is amended as follows:

PART 1—INCOME TAXES

■ **Paragraph 1.** The authority citation for part 1 continues to read in part as follows:

Authority: 26 U.S.C. 7805 * * *

■ **Par. 2.** Section 1.471–8 is revised to read as follows:

§ 1.471–8 Inventories of retail merchants.

(a) *In general.* A taxpayer that is a retail merchant may use the retail inventory method of accounting described in this section. The retail inventory method uses a formula to convert the retail selling price of ending inventory to an approximation of cost (retail cost method) or an approximation of lower of cost or market (retail LCM method). A taxpayer may use the retail inventory method instead of valuing inventory at cost under § 1.471–3 or lower of cost or market under § 1.471–4.

(b) *Computation*—(1) *In general.* A taxpayer computes the value of ending inventory under the retail inventory method by multiplying a cost complement by the retail selling prices of the goods on hand at the end of the taxable year.

(2) *Cost complement*—(i) *In general.* The cost complement is a ratio computed as follows:

(A) The numerator is the value of beginning inventory plus the cost (as determined under § 1.471–3, except as otherwise provided in this section) of goods purchased during the taxable year.

(B) The denominator is the retail selling prices of beginning inventory plus the retail selling prices of goods purchased during the year (that is, the bona fide retail selling prices of the items at the time acquired), adjusted for all permanent markups and markdowns, including markup and markdown cancellations and corrections. The denominator is not adjusted for temporary markups or markdowns.

(ii) *Vendor allowances required to reduce only cost of goods sold.* A taxpayer may not reduce the numerator of the cost complement by the amount of an allowance, discount, or price rebate that is required under § 1.471–3(e) to reduce only cost of goods sold.

(3) *Additional rules for cost complement for retail LCM method*—(i) *In general*—(A) *Margin protection payments.* A taxpayer using the retail LCM method may not reduce the numerator of the cost complement by the amount of an allowance, discount, or price rebate that is related to or intended to compensate for a permanent reduction in the taxpayer's retail selling price of inventory (a margin protection payment).

(B) *Markdowns.* A taxpayer using the retail LCM method does not adjust the denominator of the cost complement for markdowns (and markdown cancellations or corrections). Markups must be reduced by the markdowns made to cancel or correct them.

(ii) *Alternative methods for computing cost complement*—(A) *In general.* In lieu of the method described in paragraph (b)(3)(i) of this section, a taxpayer using the retail LCM method may compute the cost complement using one of the alternative methods described in this paragraph (b)(3)(ii). A taxpayer using an alternative method under this paragraph (b)(3)(ii) must use that method for all cost complements.

(B) *Adjust numerator and denominator.* A taxpayer using the retail LCM method may reduce the numerator of the cost complement by the amount of all margin protection payments if the taxpayer also reduces the denominator of the cost complement by the amount of the permanent reduction in retail selling price to which the margin protection payments relate (related markdowns).

(C) *Deemed adjustment to denominator.* A taxpayer using the retail LCM method that is able to determine the amount of all margin protection payments but cannot determine the amount of the related markdowns may reduce the numerator of the cost complement by the amount of all margin protection payments if the taxpayer also reduces the denominator by the amount that, in conjunction with the reduction of the numerator for the margin protection payments, maintains what would have been the cost complement percentage before taking into account the margin protection payment and the related markdown. A taxpayer that can determine the amount of a related markdown but not the associated margin protection payments may not use this method to compute an adjustment to the numerator.

(iii) *Statistical sampling.* A taxpayer using the retail LCM method may use statistical sampling in accordance with Rev. Proc. 2011–42 or any successor (see § 601.601(d) of this chapter), in conjunction with any method of computing the cost complement described in this paragraph (b)(3), to determine the amount of margin protection payments and related markdowns. A taxpayer using statistical sampling must use it for all margin protection payments and related markdowns associated with the inventory items valued by a particular cost complement, but is not required to use it for every cost complement.

(4) *Ending inventory retail selling prices.* A taxpayer must include all permanent markups and markdowns but may not include temporary markups or markdowns in determining the retail selling prices of goods on hand at the end of the taxable year. A taxpayer may not include a markdown that is not an actual reduction of retail selling price.

(c) *Special rules for LIFO taxpayers.* A taxpayer using the last-in, first-out (LIFO) inventory method with the retail inventory method uses the retail cost method. See § 1.472–1(k) for additional adjustments for a taxpayer using the LIFO inventory method with the retail cost method.

(d) *Scope of retail inventory method.* A taxpayer may use the retail inventory method to value ending inventory for a department, a class of goods, or a stock-keeping unit. A taxpayer maintaining more than one department or dealing in classes of goods with different percentages of gross profit must compute cost complements separately for each department or class of goods.

(e) *Examples.* The following examples illustrate the rules of this section:

Example 1. (i) R, a retail merchant who uses the retail LCM method and uses a calendar taxable year, has no beginning inventory in 2012. R purchases 40 tables during 2012 for $60 each for a total of $2,400. R offers the tables for sale at $100 each for an aggregate retail selling price of $4,000. R does not sell any tables at a price of $100, so R permanently marks down the retail selling price of its tables to $90 each. As a result of the $10 markdown, R's supplier provides R a $6 per table margin protection payment. R sells 25 tables during 2012 and has 15 tables in ending inventory at the end of 2012.

(ii) Under paragraph (b)(2)(i)(A) of this section, the numerator of the cost complement is the aggregate cost of the tables, $2,400. Under paragraph (b)(3)(i)(A) of this section, R may not reduce the numerator of the cost complement by the amount of the margin protection payment. Under paragraph (b)(2)(i)(B) of this section, the denominator of the cost complement is the aggregate of the bona fide retail selling prices of all the tables at the time acquired, $4,000. Under paragraph (b)(3)(i)(B) of this section, R does not adjust the denominator of the cost complement for the markdown. Therefore, R's cost complement is $2,400/$4,000, or 60%.

(iii) Under paragraph (b)(4) of this section, R includes the permanent markdown in determining year-end retail selling prices. Therefore, the aggregate retail selling price of R's ending table inventory is $1,350 (15 * $90). Approximating LCM under the retail method, the value of R's ending table inventory is $810 (60% * $1,350).

Example 2. (i) The facts are the same as in *Example 1*, except that R permanently reduces the retail selling price of all 40 tables to $50 per unit and the 15 tables on hand at the end of the year are marked for sale at that price. The additional $40 markdown is unrelated to a margin protection payment or other allowance.

(ii) Under paragraph (b)(3)(i)(B) of this section, R does not adjust the denominator of the cost complement for the markdown. Therefore, R's cost complement is $2,400/$4,000, or 60%.

(iii) Under paragraph (b)(4) of this section, R includes the permanent markdowns in determining year-end retail selling prices. Therefore, the aggregate retail selling price of R's ending inventory is $750 (15 * $50). Approximating LCM under the retail method, the value of R's ending inventory is $450 (60% * $750).

Example 3. (i) The facts are the same as in *Example 1*, except that R computes the cost complement using the alternative method under paragraph (b)(3)(ii)(B) of this section.

(ii) R reduces the numerator of the cost complement by the margin protection payments of $240 ($6 * 40) and reduces the denominator of the cost complement by the related markdowns of $400 ($10 * 40). Therefore, R's cost complement is $2,160/$3,600, or 60%.

(iii) Under paragraph (b)(4) of this section, R includes the permanent markdown in determining year-end retail selling prices. Therefore, the aggregate retail selling price of R's ending table inventory is $1,350 (15 * $90). Approximating LCM under the retail method, the value of R's ending inventory is $810 (60% * $1,350).

Example 4. (i) The facts are the same as in *Example 1*, except that R cannot determine the amount of its related markdowns and computes the cost complement using the alternative method under paragraph (b)(3)(ii)(C) of this section.

(ii) R reduces the numerator of the cost complement by the margin protection payments of $240 ($6 * 40). R reduces the denominator of the cost complement by the amount that, in conjunction with the reduction in the numerator, maintains the cost complement percentage before taking into account the margin protection payments and the related markdowns. R's original cost complement was 60% ($2,400/$4,000). The numerator of R's new cost complement is $2,160 ($2,400 − $240). Therefore, R reduces the denominator by $400, which maintains the cost complement of 60% ($2,160/$3,600).

(iii) Under paragraph (b)(4) of this section, R includes the permanent markdowns in determining year-end retail selling prices. Therefore, the aggregate retail selling price of R's ending table inventory is $1,350 (15 * $90). Approximating LCM under the retail method, the value of R's ending table inventory is $810 (60% * $1,350).

Example 5. (i) The facts are the same as in *Example 1*, except that R uses the LIFO inventory method. R must value inventories at cost and, under paragraph (c) of this section, uses the retail cost method.

(ii) Under paragraph (b)(2)(i)(A) of this section, R reduces the numerator of the cost complement by the amount of the margin protection payment. Under paragraph (b)(2)(i)(B) of this section, R includes the permanent markdown in the denominator of the cost complement. Therefore, R's cost complement is $2,160/$3,600, or 60%.

(iii) Under paragraph (b)(4) of this section, R includes the permanent markdown in determining year-end retail selling prices. Therefore, the aggregate retail selling price of R's ending inventory is $1,350 (15 * $90). Approximating cost under the retail method, the value of R's ending inventory is $810 (60% * $1,350).

(f) *Effective/applicability date.* This section applies to taxable years beginning after December 31, 2014. For taxable years beginning before January 1, 2015, see § 1.471–8 as contained in 26 CFR part 1, revised April 1, 2014.

John Dalrymple,
Deputy Commissioner for Services and Enforcement.

Approved: July 30, 2014

Mark J. Mazur,
Assistant Secretary of the Treasury (Tax Policy).

[FR Doc. 2014–19275 Filed 8–14–14; 8:45 am]

BILLING CODE 4830–01–P

Appendix #7
Example of a Questionnaire for the Congressmen

An example of a criteria questionnaire for Congress:

Congressional Pay inquiry form:

How many subcommittees are you assigned to? _____

How many subcommittee meeting have you attended this month? _____

How many congressional votes were you present for? _____

Were you able to read and review new bills before the vote? _____

How many constituents were you in direct contact with? _____

Did you introduce any new bills to Congress? _____

Did you take part in any unusual activities? _____

www.ingramcontent.com/pod-product-compliance
Lightning Source LLC
Chambersburg PA
CBHW030900180526
45163CB00004B/1642